A New Kind of Vegan

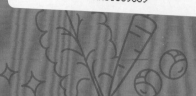

We know what you're thinking: Vegan food is bland, vegan food isn't satisfying, vegan food is, well, crunchy. We feel you—but now's the time to leave those dusty preconceived notions at the door. **We spent countless hours dreaming up vegan recipes with a different approach: flavor first.** Whether you're a lifelong vegan or a curious omnivore, you're guaranteed to find a new weeknight dinner, colorful salad, or comforting soup.

First off: Eating vegan shouldn't have to feel like a sacrifice. So we took inspiration from our favorite meat–based dishes—did you really think we'd deprive ourselves of buffalo wings?! Our tempeh rendition (p. 95) is just as saucy, spicy, and satisfying as the real thing. And date night will feel extra-special when grilled Eggplant "Steak" Frites with Chimichurri (p. 156) or king trumpet mushroom "scallops" with corn succotash (p. 154) is on the menu.

We also explored some quintessential naturally vegan dishes from around the world, inspiring recipes like our herb–packed baked falafel with minty tahini dip (p. 86), ultra–comforting South Asian Khichdi (p. 112), and the Mayan dip Sikil Pa'k (p. 18) that spotlights the enticing flavor of smoky toasted pepitas.

I've never followed a strict vegan diet, but as the daughter of organic farmers and former vegetarians, meat has never played a big role in my life. I learned early to shed conventional stereotypes and allowed myself to play with and personalize recipes, opening up a whole new world of plant-based eating. Vegan food might be saddled with an uptight reputation, but the recipes in this book prove that the only real barrier is your own creativity.

Happy cooking,
Lena Abraham, Delish Senior Food Editor

Contents

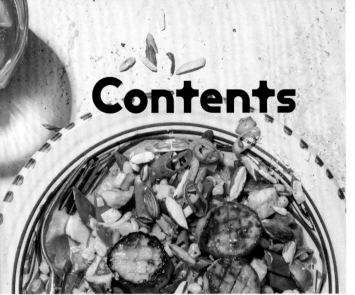

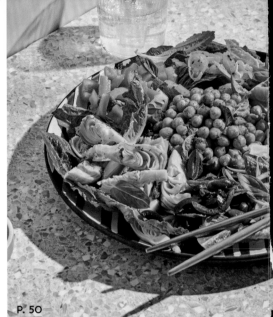

P. 50

CHAPTER 2:
MIGHTY SALADS

Summer Panzanella	34
Taco Salad	37
Avocado & Tomato Salad	38
Coconut Ranch Kale Salad	41
Lentil Salad	42
Moroccan Carrot Salad	45
Classic Shallot Vinaigrette	46
Creamy Noodle Salad	49
Antipasto Chopped Salad	50
Jerk Tofu Grain Bowl	52
Super Green Pasta Salad	56

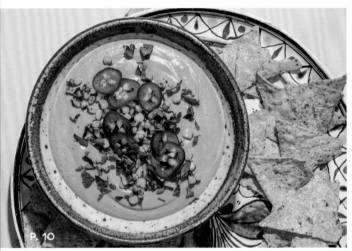

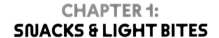

P. 10

CHAPTER 1:
SNACKS & LIGHT BITES

Chipotle "Queso"	10
Classic Bruschetta	13
Muhammara	14
Scallion Pancakes	17
Sikil P'ak	18
The Perfect Snack Board	20
Curry–Lime Cashews	23
Garlicky Citrus Marinated Beans	24
Avocado Hummus	27
Rosemary Focaccia	28
Ssamjang	31

CHAPTER 3: BEST-EVER SOUPS

White Bean & Kale Soup	60
French Onion Lentil Stew	63
Tortilla Soup	64
Curried Butternut Squash Soup	67
Red Miso Veggie Ramen	68
Carrot & Coriander Soup	71
New England "Clam" Chowder	72
Gazpacho	75
Chickpea Noodle Soup	76

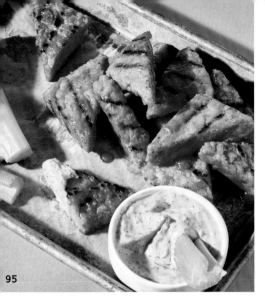

95

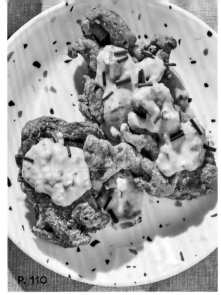

P. 110

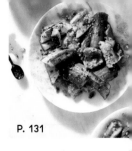

P. 131

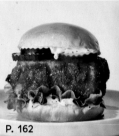

P. 162

CHAPTER 4: EASY WEEKNIGHTS

Chipotle Lentil Tacos	80
Tofu Bánh Mì	82
Seitan "Lomo" Saltado	84
Herby Baked Falafel with Spicy Mint Tahini Dip	86
Chickpea "Tuna" Salad	88
Extra Lemony Seitan Piccata	91
Tempeh & Broccoli Rabe Orecchiette	92
Tempeh Buffalo "Wings"	95

CHAPTER 5: COMFORT FOOD

Creamy Mac & "Cheese"	98
"Meatloaf" & Sesame Mashed Potatoes	100
BBQ Cauliflower Pizza	102
Cashew Cream Alfredo	105
Sesame Tofu Katsu Curry	106
Chicken-Fried Mushrooms & Gravy	110
Spiced Khichdi	112
Best-Ever Chickpea "Meatballs"	115
Cincinnati-Style Chili Dogs	116
Chipotle "Queso" Crunchy Wraps	118
BBQ Tempeh Sandwiches	120

CHAPTER 6: EXTRA VEGGIES

Mushroom "Calamari" with Spicy Marinara	124
Ratatouille	127
Kung Pao Brussels Sprouts	128
Chili Oil Smashed Cucumbers	131
Sichuan-Style "Fish Fragrant" Eggplant	132
Giardiniera	134
BBQ Braised Kale	136
Chili Garlic Fried Cauliflower	139
Miso Maple Glazed Carrots	140
Butternut Squash Potstickers	142
Gamja Jorim	144

CHAPTER 7: WEEKENDS & SPECIAL OCCASIONS

Polenta with Wild Mushroom Ragu	148
Chipotle Tofu & Pineapple Skewers	150
Veggie Paella (Paella Verdura)	152
Seared "Scallops" & Corn Succotash	154
Eggplant "Steak" Frites with Chimichurri	156
Mushroom Pot Pie	158
Spicy Fried "Chicken" Sandwich	162
Whole Roasted Cabbage	164
Charred Lemon-Asparagus Risotto	166

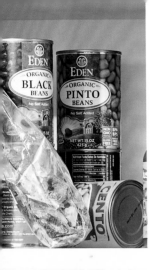

Vegan Kitchen Essentials

With a well-stocked pantry and a few simple tools, plant-based cooking is a breeze. These are the ingredients we keep on hand so an improvised meal or snack is always within reach.

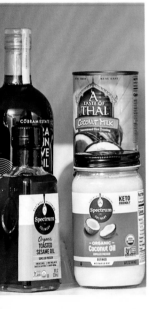

Nutritional Yeast
With lots of cheesy, umami flavor, these yellow flakes are great as a finishing touch, or stirred into sauces like in our Cashew Cream Alfredo on p. 105.

Maple Syrup & Agave
Counteract bitter and sour flavors with these natural sweeteners.

Vegetable Broth
Not just for soups and stews! Use this to add flavor while cooking dried beans or grains; we're especially fond of long-lasting and compact vegan bouillon cubes.

Whole Spices
For deeper, more complex flavor that lasts longer on the shelf, buy whole spices and grind them in a spice or coffee grinder or with a mortar and pestle.

Dried Mushrooms
Major umami bombs, these bring a distinctly meaty flavor to everything from velvety gravies and rich pot pies.

Nuts & Seeds
Great for adding protein and crunch. Use as a mix-in, a garnish, or pureed into a sauce or dip, like our Sikil P'ak on p. 18.

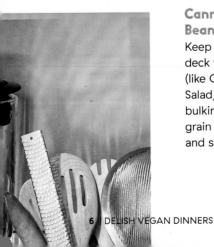

Canned or Dried Beans
Keep a variety on deck for quick meals (like Chickpea "Tuna" Salad, p. 88) and bulking up salads, grain bowls, soups, and skillet dinners.

Oils
Extra-virgin is an obvious choice, but it's good to have flavored oils for finishing (like toasted sesame) and some with neutral flavor that can handle high heat cooking, like vegetable, peanut, or grapeseed.

Miso
This Japanese fermented paste is often soy-based, but there are countless alternatives. White miso is the mildest, but it still gives a big boost of savory flavor to soups, stews, sauces, and more.

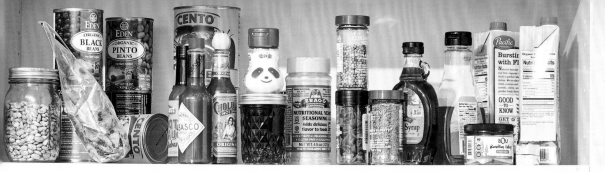

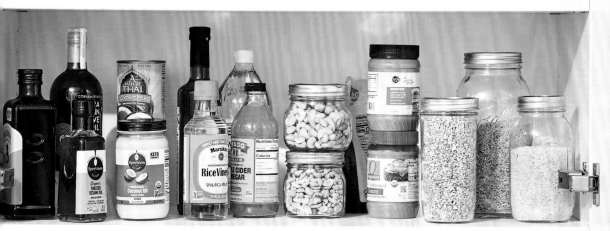

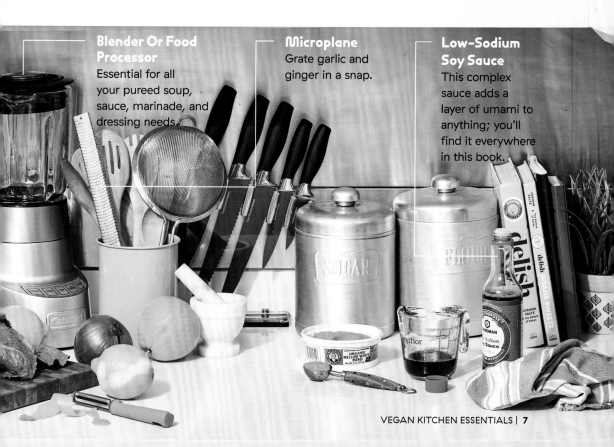

Blender Or Food Processor
Essential for all your pureed soup, sauce, marinade, and dressing needs.

Microplane
Grate garlic and ginger in a snap.

Low-Sodium Soy Sauce
This complex sauce adds a layer of umami to anything; you'll find it everywhere in this book.

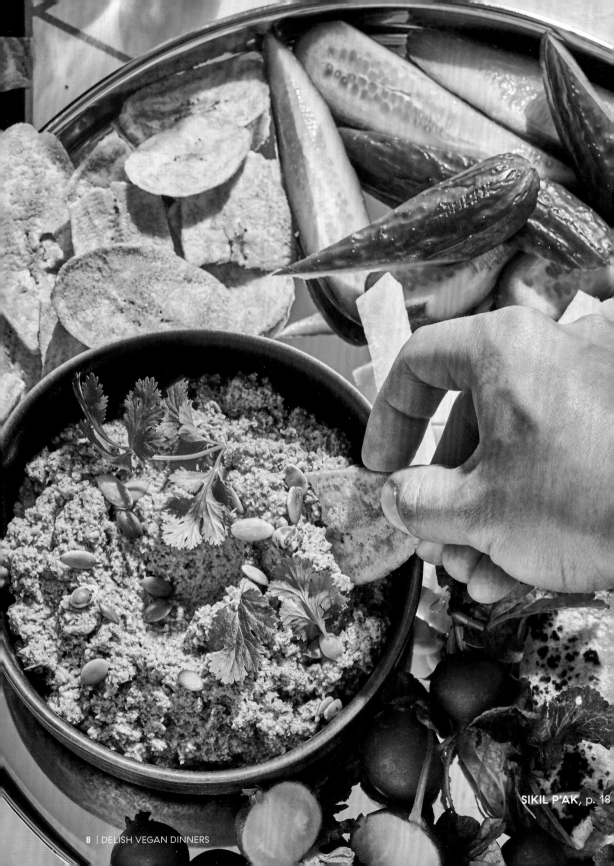

SIKIL P'AK, p. 18

CHAPTER ONE

SNACKS & LIGHT BITES

Everything you need for some Grade-A grazing.

Chipotle "Queso"

The infinitely versatile cashew does it again with this "cheesy" Tex–Mex dip that's hard to distinguish from the original. Make it yours: Swap the chipotle with your favorite salsa, a can of Ro–tel, or harissa for a slightly different flavor profile.

2 cups raw cashews (10 ounces)

3½ teaspoons chili powder, divided

4 teaspoons chipotle en adobo sauce, divided

1 clove garlic

1 teaspoon nutritional yeast

1 teaspoon onion powder

½ teaspoon ground turmeric

½ teaspoon garlic powder

½ teaspoon ground cumin

1½ cups boiling water, plus more as needed

Kosher salt

2 tablespoons extra-virgin olive oil

1 cup fresh or frozen thawed corn

½ jalapeño, thinly sliced

Cilantro leaves, for garnish

Tortilla chips, for serving

1. Fill a blender with cashews, 2½ teaspoons chili powder, 3 teaspoons chipotle sauce, garlic, nutritional yeast, onion powder, turmeric, garlic powder, and cumin. Carefully pour boiling water into blender. Cover and blend on high until smooth, about 1 minute. Season with salt and add extra water by the tablespoon as needed to thin to a queso consistency. Blend until combined. Transfer queso into a serving bowl.

2. Heat a medium skillet over medium-high and add oil and corn. Cook, stirring until lightly charred, about 1 to 2 minutes. Remove from heat and stir in remaining teaspoon of chile powder and remaining teaspoon of chipotle sauce. Spoon corn over center of "queso," scatter jalapeño and cilantro on top, and serve with tortilla chips.

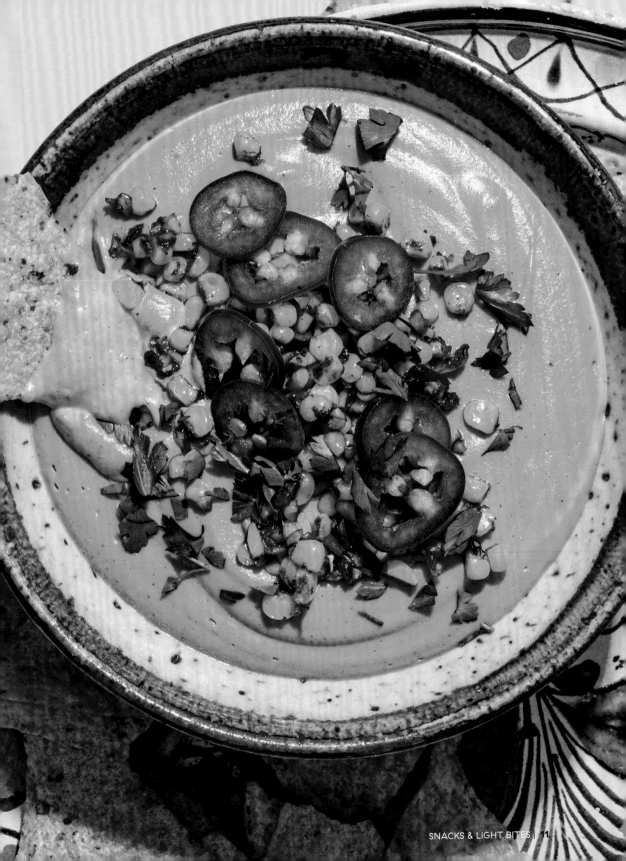

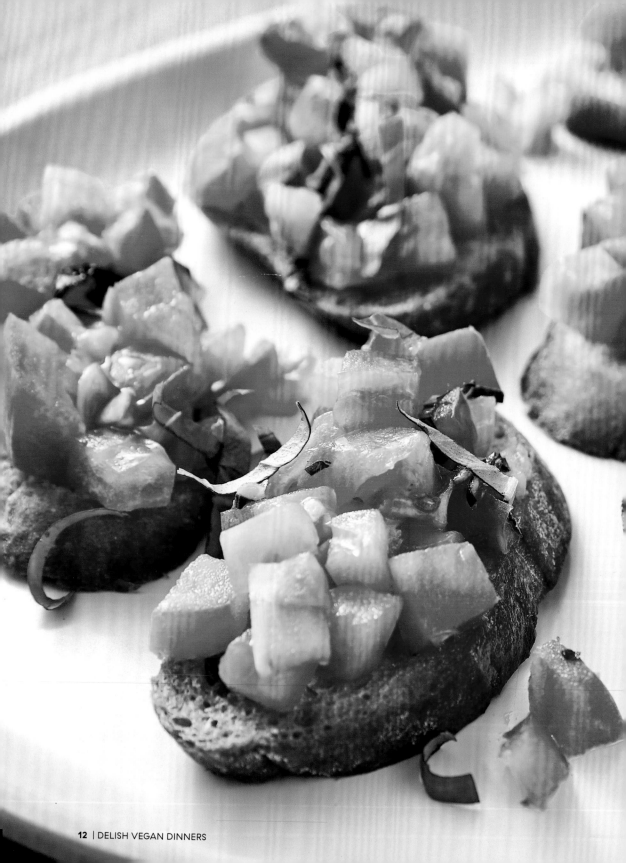

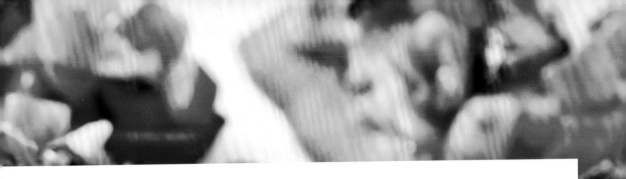

Classic Bruschetta

 SERVES 10 | **TOTAL TIME: 50 MIN**

This juicy, flavorful appetizer proves that sometimes simple is best. Beyond summertime, go for cherry or grape tomatoes; these varieties taste best out of season.

¼ cup extra-virgin olive oil, plus more for brushing

4 cloves garlic, 2 thinly sliced and 2 halved, divided

4 large tomatoes, diced

¼ cup thinly sliced basil

2 tablespoons balsamic vinegar

1 teaspoon kosher salt

Pinch of crushed red pepper flakes

1 large baguette, sliced ¼ inch thick on bias

1. Make marinated tomatoes: In a medium skillet over medium-low heat, heat oil. Add garlic and cook until lightly golden, 2 to 4 minutes, then remove from heat and let cool.

2. In a large bowl, toss together tomatoes, basil, vinegar, salt, and red pepper flakes. Add garlic and oil from skillet and toss to combine. Let marinate for at least 30 minutes.

3. Meanwhile, toast bread: Preheat oven to 400°F. Lightly brush bread on both sides with oil and place on large baking sheet. Toast bread until golden, 10 to 15 minutes, turning halfway through. Let bread cool for 5 minutes, then rub tops of bread with halved garlic cloves.

4. Spoon tomatoes on top of bread just before serving.

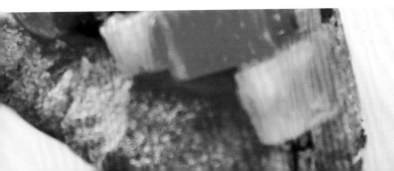
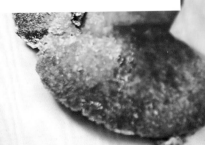

Muhammara

 SERVES 4 | 🕐 **TOTAL TIME: 55 MIN**

Popular throughout the Middle East but originally from Syria, this dip is sweet, smoky, and spicy all in one. Pomegranate molasses is integral to a classic muhammara and is sold at most major grocery stores, but a drizzle of agave and squeeze of citrus can stand in for its sweet tanginess.

2 red bell peppers
2 slices bread, preferably white
  or sourdough
½ cup walnuts
Juice of ½ lemon
2 teaspoons Aleppo pepper
½ teaspoon ground paprika
1 clove garlic
1 tablespoon pomegranate
  molasses
3 tablespoons extra-virgin olive oil
Kosher salt
Freshly ground black pepper

1. Roast peppers by placing over a flame of a gas burner until well charred all over, about 2 minutes per side. Alternatively, cut peppers in half and remove stem and seeds. Place cut-side down on a parchment-lined baking sheet and bake at 475°F until peppers are well charred, about 30 minutes.

2. Place peppers immediately into a large bowl and cover tightly with plastic wrap. Let steam for 10 minutes. Remove from bowl and peel off charred skin. It should fall off easily, but you can use the back of your knife to help. Discard skin, seeds, and stem. Slice peppers.

3. Preheat oven to 300°F. Tear bread to fit into a food processor, then pulse into rough bread crumbs. Measure out ¾ cup bread crumbs and spread out on a small baking sheet. Bake until dried out, about 10 minutes. Wipe out food processor and save any extra bread crumbs for another use.

4. Place walnuts on another small baking sheet and bake until toasted and fragrant, about 15 minutes.

5. Add roasted bell peppers, bread crumbs, toasted walnuts, lemon juice, Aleppo, paprika, garlic, and pomegranate molasses to food processor and blend until well combined. With motor running, slowly add oil. Season with salt and pepper.

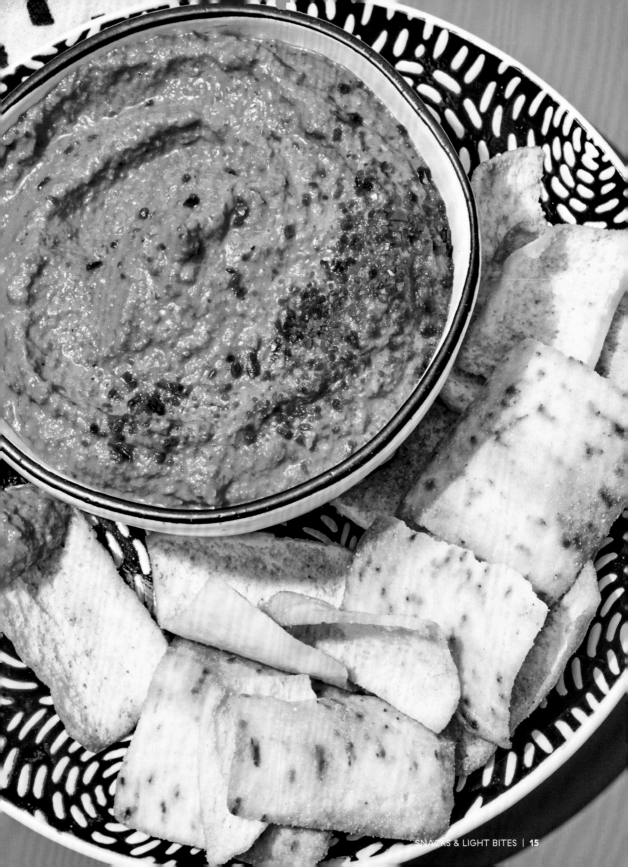

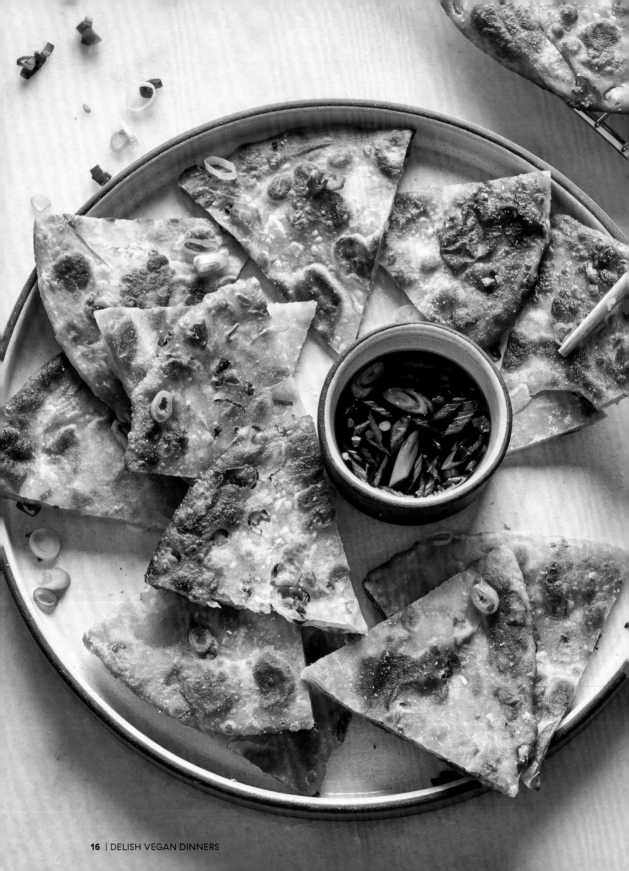

Scallion Pancakes

 SERVES 4 | **TOTAL TIME: 45 MIN**

Crispy, flaky, and slightly chewy, these scallion pancakes never disappoint. Make sure to keep your dough covered so it stays hydrated and easily workable.

FOR THE PANCAKES

2 cups all-purpose flour
1 cup boiling water
¼ cup plus 2 tablespoons
   vegetable oil, divided
2 tablespoons sesame oil
1 cup thinly sliced scallions,
   from about 4 whole scallions
Kosher salt

FOR THE DIPPING SAUCE

2 tablespoons rice wine vinegar
2 tablespoons low-sodium soy
   sauce
1 scallion, thinly sliced
Pinch of crushed red pepper
   flakes (optional)
Kosher salt

1. Combine flour and boiling water in a large bowl and stir to combine until a mass of dough forms. Transfer dough to a lightly floured surface and knead until smooth, slightly tacky ball forms, 3 to 4 minutes.

2. Transfer dough ball to a medium bowl and cover with a kitchen towel or plastic wrap. Let rest 30 minutes at room temperature, or up to overnight in fridge.

3. Meanwhile, mix 2 tablespoons vegetable oil and sesame oil in a small bowl.

4. Make dipping sauce: In a small bowl, stir together vinegar, soy sauce, scallions, and pepper flakes (if usng).

5. Separate dough into 4 equal balls. Return 3 to bowl and recover with kitchen towel or plastic wrap. Roll remaining ball into an 8-inch disk, and brush with a thin layer of oil mixture. Roll tightly into a cylinder then twist into a tight spiral (like a cinnamon roll), tucking outer end underneath roll. Using palm of your hand, flatten spiral, then roll out again into an 8-inch disk. Brush top with another thin layer of oil and scatter with ¼ cup sliced scallions. Roll up disk again then roll into spiral. Roll into an 8-inch disk then repeat with remaining dough balls.

6. Add remaining ¼ cup vegetable oil to an 8-inch skillet over medium-high heat until shimmering and gently add first pancake. Cook, undisturbed, until golden on one side. Flip and cook until golden on underside, about 2 to 3 minutes per side. Remove to paper towel-lined plate and season immediately with salt. Repeat with remaining pancakes, adding more oil if necessary.

7. Cut pancakes into triangles and serve with dipping sauce.

Sikil P'ak

If salsa verde and hummus had a kid, it would remind us of this dip. Our take on Sikil p'ak, which in Mayan means "pumpkin seed" and "tomato," is inspired by the Yucatecan version. We use hulled pepitas and charred tomatillos, and its subtle smokiness keeps us coming back for more.

¾ cup plus 1 tablespoon hulled raw pepitas (about 5 ounces)

4 tomatillos, husks removed and rinsed (about 6 ounces)

2 shallots, peeled (about 3 ounces)

2 cloves garlic, peeled

1 jalapeño, stem removed

2 cups cilantro, leaves and tender stems roughly chopped, plus leaves for garnish

¼ cup fresh lime juice (from about 3 limes)

2 teaspoons lime zest

1 teaspoon kosher salt, plus more to taste

TO SERVE

Sliced cucumbers, radishes, raw jicama sticks, corn tortillas, or plantain chips

1. In a medium skillet over medium-high heat, toast pepitas until lightly browned, 5 minutes, stirring frequently. Set aside 1 tablespoon for garnish and transfer remaining into a food processor. Process for about 30 seconds until finely ground. It should look like wet sand.

2. In same skillet over medium-high heat, add tomatillos, shallots, garlic, and jalapeño. Using tongs, flip each as needed and transfer into food processor when charred on all sides.

3. Add cilantro, lime juice and zest, and salt into food processor. Pulse about 20 times until cilantro is fully incorporated then process until charred vegetables are coarsely chopped, scraping down sides as needed. Taste and adjust seasoning with salt and lime juice. It should taste nutty, limey, and herby. Transfer to a bowl and garnish with reserved pepitas and cilantro leaves. Serve with suggested crudités.

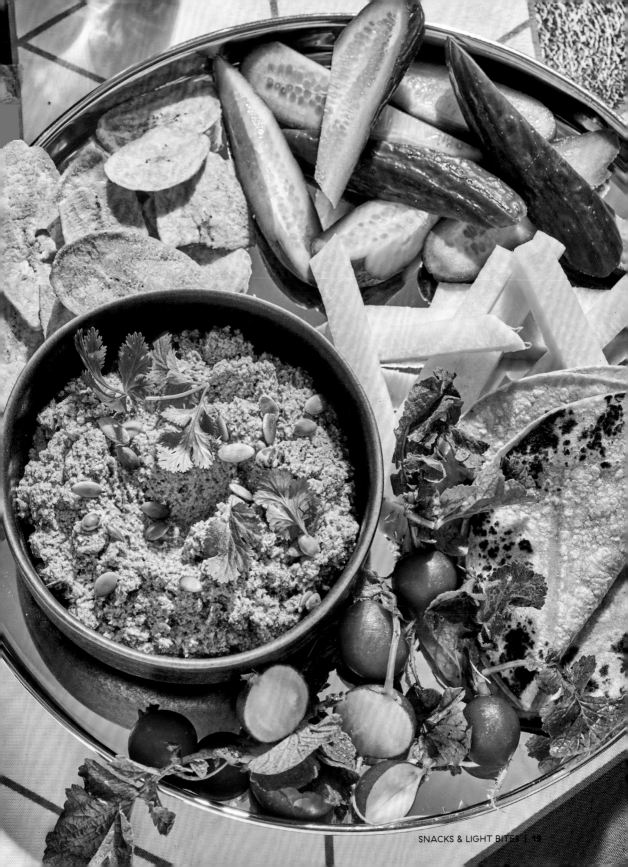

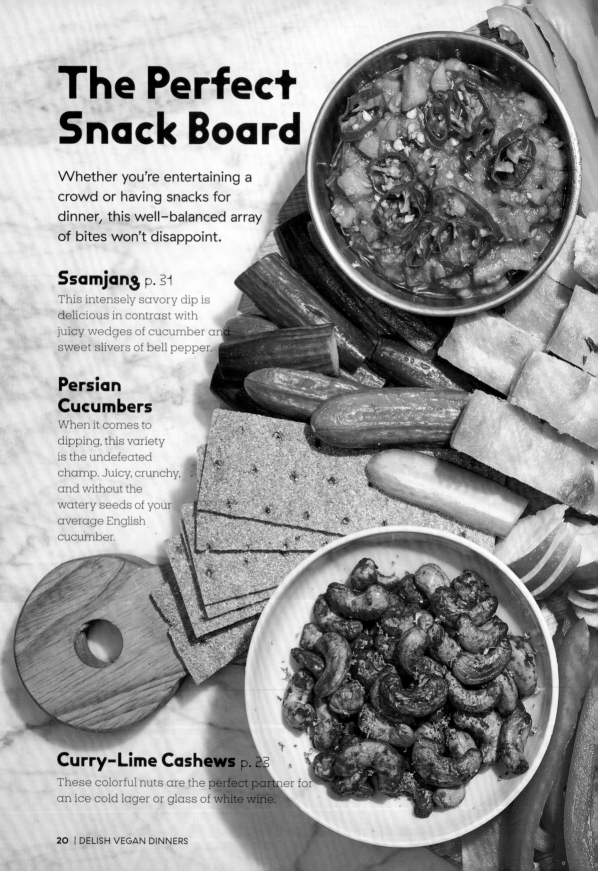

The Perfect Snack Board

Whether you're entertaining a crowd or having snacks for dinner, this well-balanced array of bites won't disappoint.

Ssamjang p. 31

This intensely savory dip is delicious in contrast with juicy wedges of cucumber and sweet slivers of bell pepper.

Persian Cucumbers

When it comes to dipping, this variety is the undefeated champ. Juicy, crunchy, and without the watery seeds of your average English cucumber.

Curry-Lime Cashews p. 23

These colorful nuts are the perfect partner for an ice cold lager or glass of white wine.

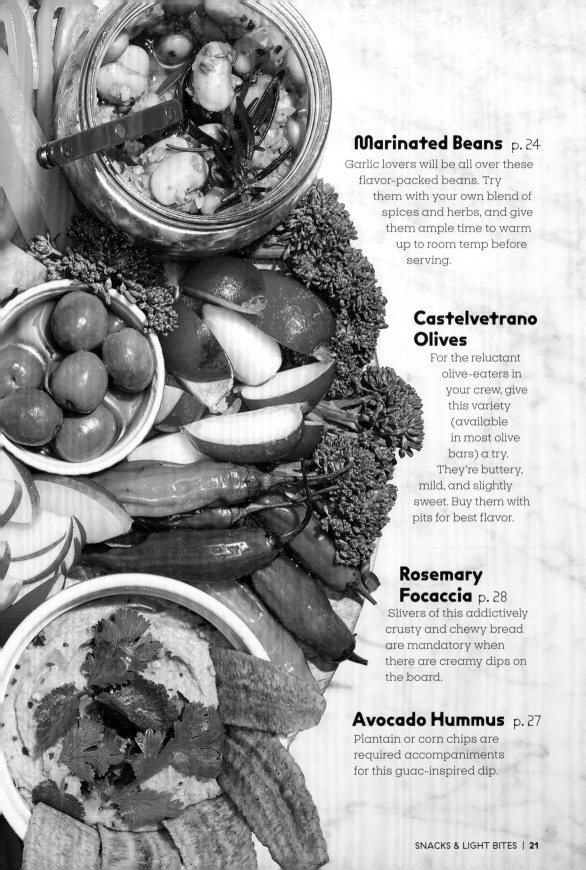

Marinated Beans p. 24

Garlic lovers will be all over these flavor-packed beans. Try them with your own blend of spices and herbs, and give them ample time to warm up to room temp before serving.

Castelvetrano Olives

For the reluctant olive-eaters in your crew, give this variety (available in most olive bars) a try. They're buttery, mild, and slightly sweet. Buy them with pits for best flavor.

Rosemary Focaccia p. 28

Slivers of this addictively crusty and chewy bread are mandatory when there are creamy dips on the board.

Avocado Hummus p. 27

Plantain or corn chips are required accompaniments for this guac-inspired dip.

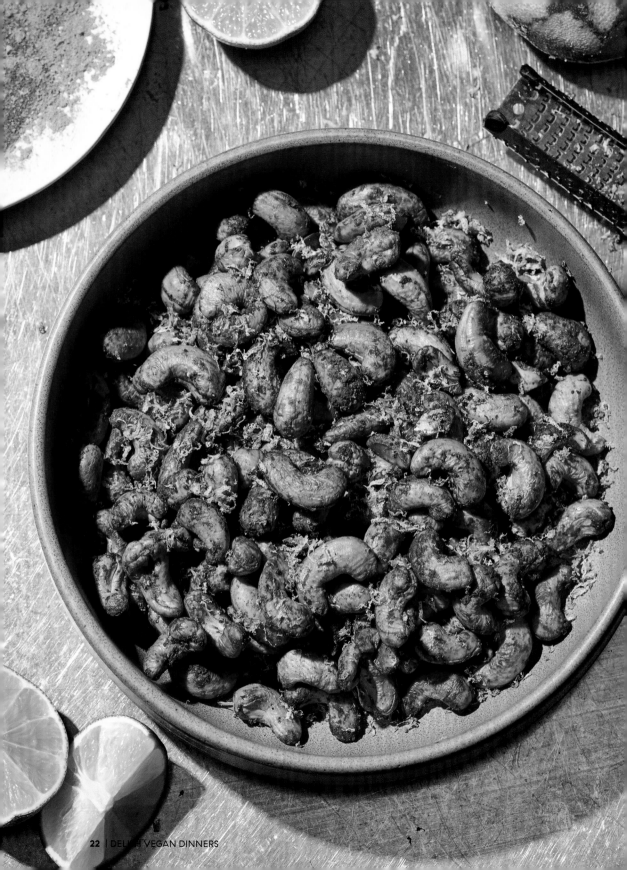

Curry-Lime Cashews

 MAKES 2 CUPS | **TOTAL TIME: 40 MIN**

Sure, a handful of these nuts curbs hunger pangs, but they're more than just a snack. For some crunch, try them chopped up on your favorite roasted vegetables along with a spoonful of dairy-free yogurt.

2 cups raw cashews (10 ounces)
1 tablespoon extra-virgin olive oil
Kosher salt
1 tablespoon yellow curry powder
2 teaspoons granulated sugar
½ teaspoon ground turmeric
¼ teaspoon sweet paprika
Freshly ground black pepper
3 tablespoons fresh lime juice,
    plus 1 lime finely zested

1. Preheat oven to 300°F. Line a rimmed baking sheet with parchment paper. Pour cashews onto prepared baking sheet and toss with oil and ¼ teaspoon salt. Spread into an even layer. Bake until cashews are light golden, tossing halfway through, about 15 minutes.

2. Meanwhile, in a small bowl, whisk curry powder, sugar, turmeric, paprika, and a pinch of black pepper with lime juice until smooth.

3. Remove tray from oven and carefully pour spice mixture over cashews; toss well to coat cashews and spread into an even layer.

4. Return tray to oven and bake about 15 minutes more, tossing halfway through, until cashews are toasted and curry mixture bakes into cashews (they will appear to lose their crispiness but will crisp back up as they cool) and turns just slightly darker in color.

5. Scrape cashews off hot sheet tray onto a plate in an even layer and sprinkle with salt and lime zest. Let cool at least 15 minutes and serve warm or cool completely and serve at room temperature.

Garlicky Citrus Marinated Beans

 SERVES 4 | **TOTAL TIME: 1 HR 10 MIN**

Keep a jar of these addictive marinated beans in your fridge and have a snack on deck at all times. They're also an instant meal-maker; we love them stirred into farro or quinoa for a quick grain salad, topped on toast with roasted veggies, or folded into freshly boiled pasta and sautéed greens.

1 small shallot, minced

3 tablespoons white wine vinegar

Kosher salt

1 (15-ounce) can chickpeas, white beans, or black-eyed peas

2 (2-inch) pieces orange or lemon peel

4 (2-inch) sprigs fresh rosemary

1 garlic clove, grated

½ cup extra-virgin olive oil

1 to 1½ teaspoons crushed red pepper flakes, depending on heat preference

½ teaspoon cumin seeds, crushed

½ teaspoon fennel seeds, crushed

1. Combine minced shallot and white wine vinegar in a medium bowl and season with a pinch of salt. Stir to combine and set aside.

2. Combine beans, citrus peel, rosemary, and garlic in a heatproof bowl.

3. Combine oil, red pepper flakes, cumin seeds, and fennel seeds in a small pot over medium heat. When small bubbles form on spices, cook, stirring frequently, for 30 seconds, until spices are fragrant and have darkened slightly in color. Pour over beans and stir to coat.

4. Stir shallot mixture into bean mixture. Transfer to a resealable container (a 16-ounce glass jar is perfect for this) and let marinate at least 1 hour, turning container occasionally.

PRO TIP! Beans will last in the refrigerator for 1 week. If the oil solidifies, set them out at room temperature for 15 minutes, then stir before serving.

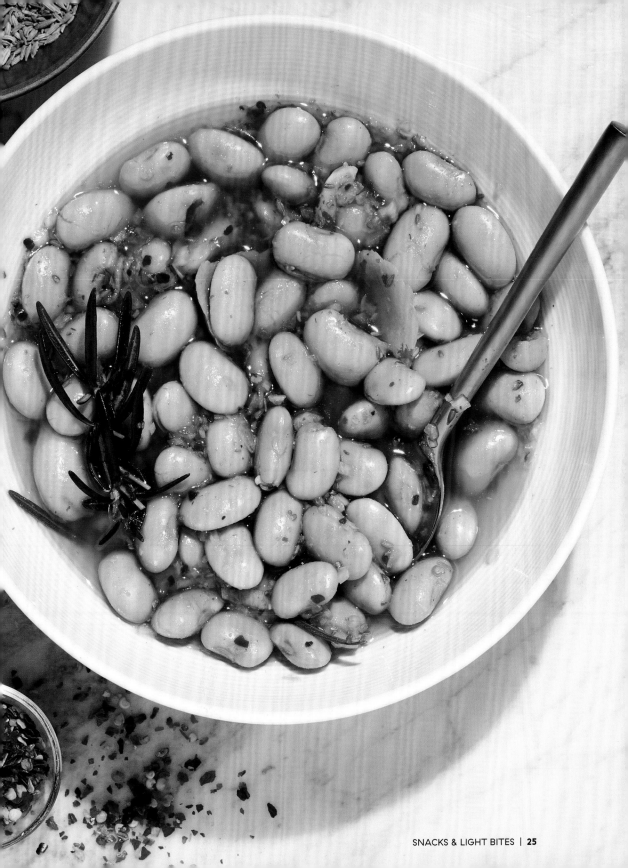

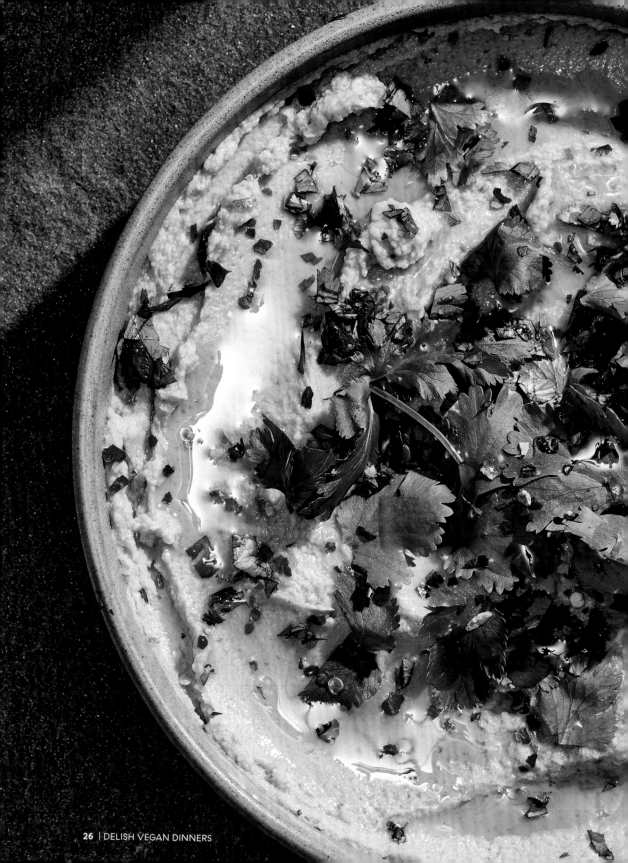

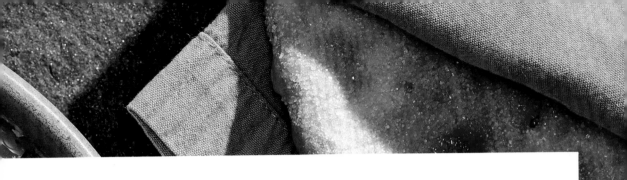

Avocado Hummus

🍴 **SERVES 6-8** | ⓛ **TOTAL TIME: 10 MIN** |

This hummus takes inspiration from guacamole for a creamy–tart snack that you can eat with veggies or chips or as a spread. For an herbier version, throw ¼ cup chopped cilantro into the food processor as you blend it up.

2 cups canned chickpeas, drained and rinsed
2 ripe avocados, peeled and cored
⅓ cup tahini
¼ cup fresh lime juice
2 cloves garlic
3 tablespoons olive oil, plus more for serving
1 teaspoon cumin
Kosher salt
1 tablespoon chopped cilantro, for garnish
Red pepper flakes, for garnish

1. Combine chickpeas, avocados, tahini, lime juice, garlic, olive oil, and cumin in bowl of a food processor and season with salt. Blend until smooth.

2. Transfer mixture to serving bowl and garnish with cilantro and red pepper flakes. Drizzle with more olive oil and serve.

Rosemary Focaccia

 SERVES 20   **TOTAL TIME: 1 HR 40 MIN**

If you're new to yeasted bread baking, this focaccia is a great place to start. Rosemary is a classic topping, but don't feel the need to stop there. Sesame seeds, sun-dried tomatoes, olives, caramelized onions, or roasted red peppers are all A+ additions.

1¼ cups water

1 teaspoon granulated sugar

1 (0.25-ounce) packet (or 2¼ teaspoons) active dry yeast

½ cup extra-virgin olive oil, divided

3¼ cups all-purpose flour, plus more as needed

2 teaspoons kosher salt

2 tablespoons fresh rosemary leaves

Flaky sea salt

1. Bloom yeast: To a small, microwave-safe bowl or glass measuring cup, add water. Microwave until lukewarm, about 40 seconds. Add sugar and stir to dissolve, then sprinkle yeast over top and stir to combine. Let sit until frothy, about 15 minutes.

2. Make dough: Grease a large bowl with 2 tablespoons olive oil. In another large bowl, add flour, salt, and 2 more tablespoons olive oil. Pour in yeast mixture, then mix with a wooden spoon until everything is combined. Knead against side of bowl until dough comes together in a loose ball. Transfer to a lightly floured work surface and knead until elastic and smooth, about 5 minutes. Transfer to greased bowl and toss to coat dough in oil. Cover with plastic wrap and let rise until doubled in size, about 1 hour.

3. Toward end of rise, preheat oven to 400°F. Evenly grease a 9x13-inch baking sheet with 2 more tablespoons olive oil. Lightly punch down dough to deflate slightly then transfer to prepared baking sheet. Press with your fingers to stretch and guide dough to edges of sheet, making indentations all over as you go. Drizzle top with 2 more tablespoons olive oil and brush to coat then sprinkle all over with rosemary and flaky salt. (For an even crunchier golden top, feel free to use more olive oil!)

4. Bake until focaccia is puffy and golden, about 25 minutes.

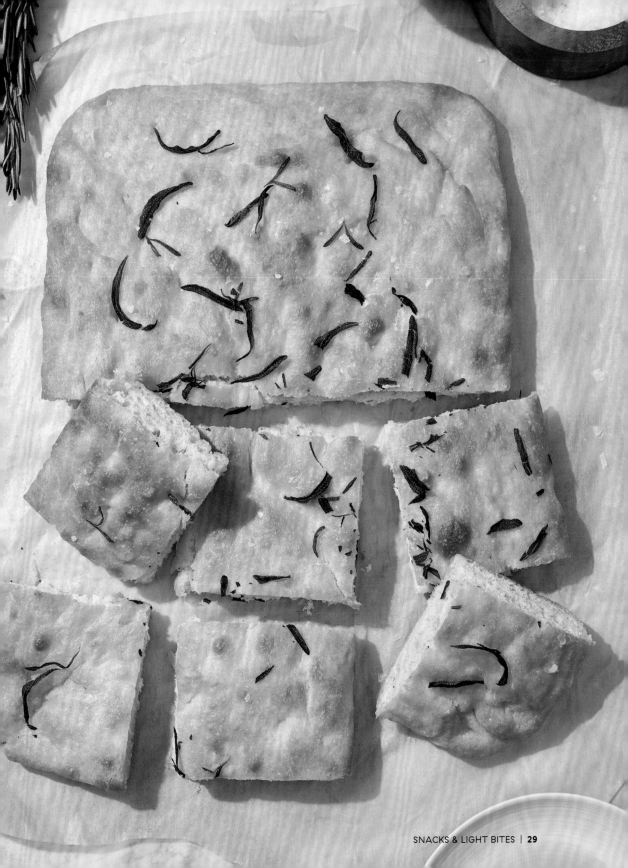

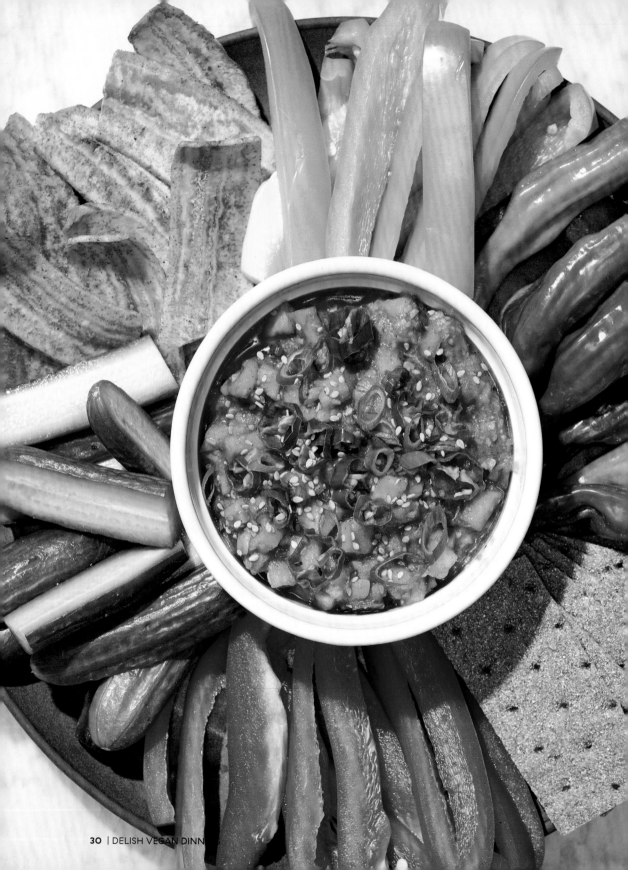

Ssamjang

🍴 SERVES 4–6	TOTAL TIME: 10 MIN

Arrange a smorgasbord of all the crunchy veggies you can get your hands on, because we know a spicy–funky–salty–sweet–creamy–crunchy dip that will keep you coming back for more. It's called *ssamjang*—technically not a dip but a *jang* (paste) that Koreans dollop in *ssam* (a wrap), with grilled meat and crisp greens. This slightly chunky version is sweetened with agave syrup and tiny bites of apple.

⅓ cup doenjang (fermented Korean soybean paste)

1 tablespoon gochujang (fermented Korean chile paste)

1 tablespoon agave syrup

1 tablespoon plus 1 teaspoon sesame oil

2 teaspoons toasted sesame seeds

1 small apple (Honeycrisp, Gala, or Fuji), peeled, cored, and finely diced (about 1 cup)

2 shishito peppers, thinly sliced into rounds

1 clove garlic, minced

1 scallion, thinly sliced

1. In a small bowl, stir doenjang, gochujang, agave syrup, sesame oil, sesame seeds, apple, shishito peppers, garlic, and scallion until combined. Serve with suggested crudités.

PRO TIP!

We love serving this dip with...everything. Our favorite dippers to try: sliced cucumbers, radishes, endive, pepper or sesame or rice crackers.

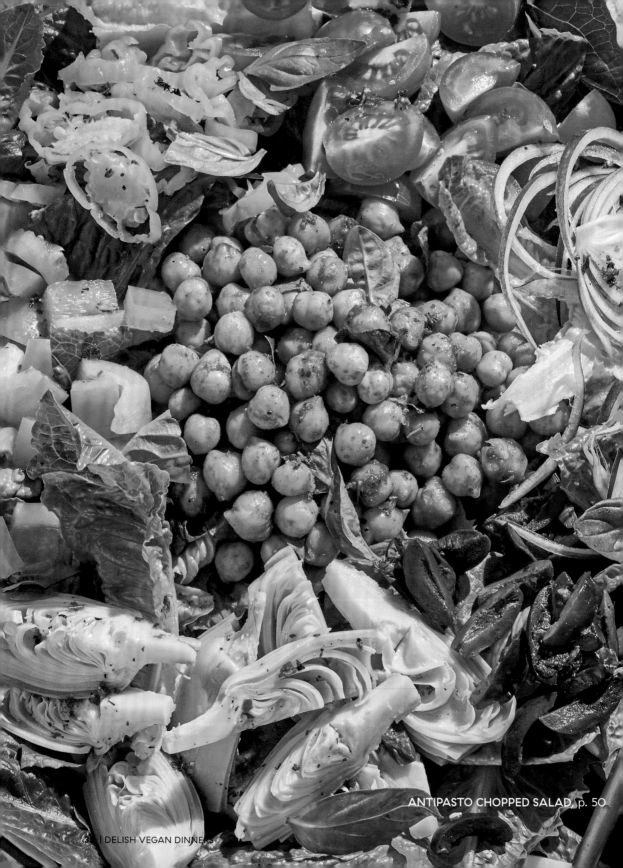

ANTIPASTO CHOPPED SALAD, p. 50

CHAPTER TWO

MIGHTY SALADS

Eating your greens has never been so easy.

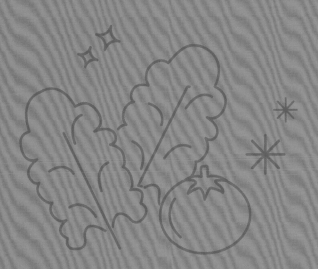

Summer Panzanella

The best time to make this salad is right in the heat of summer, when tomatoes are at their sweetest. Throw in some chopped avocado or toasted nuts for a heartier version.

2 large baguettes, cut into 1-inch cubes

½ cup extra-virgin olive oil, divided

3 tablespoons red wine vinegar

1 teaspoon agave syrup

Kosher salt

Freshly ground black pepper

1 large seedless cucumber, roughly chopped

2 pints cherry tomatoes (preferably multicolored), halved

1 red onion, chopped

1 clove garlic, minced

1 bunch basil, torn

1. Preheat a large skillet over medium-high heat.

2. In a large bowl, toss bread with ¼ cup olive oil. Add bread to skillet and toast until golden and crisp, about 10 minutes. Drain and set aside to cool.

3. Make dressing: In a small bowl, whisk together red wine vinegar, remaining ¼ cup olive oil, and agave. Season with salt and pepper.

4. To large bowl, add crispy bread, cucumber, tomatoes, onion, and garlic. Toss with dressing until evenly coated and season with more salt and pepper.

5. Garnish with basil and serve.

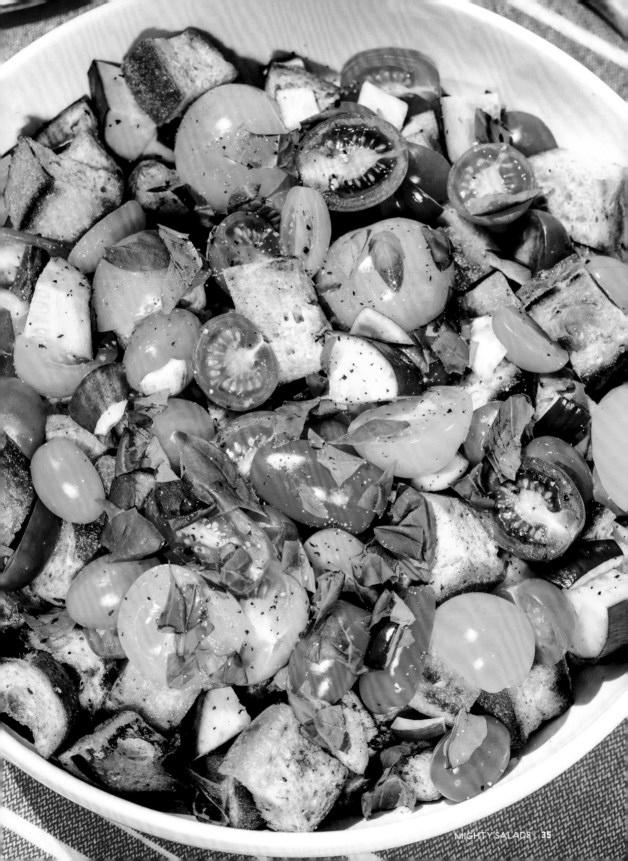

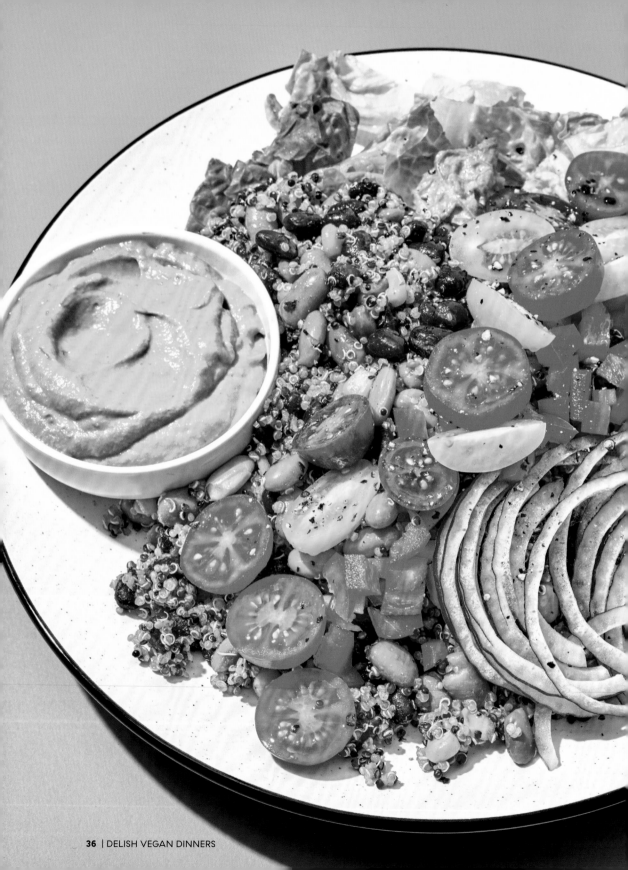

Taco Salad

 SERVES 6 | 🕐 **TOTAL TIME: 40 MIN**

Fresh, crunchy, and full of healthy ingredients, this hearty salad will keep you going for hours. If meal prep is your goal, hold off on mixing in the dressing and lettuce to keep the salad fresh longer.

FOR THE SALAD

2 cups water

1 cup quinoa

1 (15-ounce) can black beans, rinsed and drained

1 (15-ounce) can pinto beans, rinsed and drained

1 cup corn

1 tablespoon taco seasoning

Kosher salt

Freshly ground black pepper

Chopped romaine

½ small red onion, thinly sliced

1 cup cherry tomatoes, halved

1 bell pepper, chopped

Tortilla chips

FOR THE DRESSING

2 large avocados, pitted

1 chipotle in adobo sauce, plus 1 teaspoon sauce

Juice of 1 lime

¼ cup fresh cilantro

2 cloves garlic

¼ cup water

3 tablespoons extra-virgin olive oil

2 tablespoons white wine vinegar

Kosher salt

Freshly ground black pepper

1. In a medium pot over medium heat, bring water to a boil. Add quinoa, reduce heat to a simmer, then cover and cook 12 minutes, or until water is absorbed. Remove from heat but keep covered for 10 minutes.

2. Add beans, corn, and taco seasoning to warm quinoa and toss to combine. Season with salt and pepper.

3. In a blender or small food processor, blend together dressing ingredients. Season with salt and pepper. Add more vinegar or water to thin dressing as desired.

4. In a large bowl, add romaine and toss with quinoa mixture, red onions, tomatoes, and bell pepper. Serve with chipotle dressing and tortilla chips on the side.

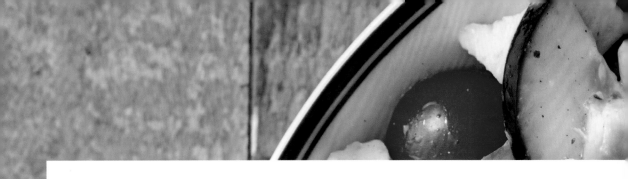

Avocado & Tomato Salad

 SERVES 4 | **TOTAL TIME: 10 MIN**

This summery salad works as a light side, or as a dip with tortilla chips. For a layer of smoky flavor, grill or sear your corn first!

¼ cup extra-virgin olive oil
Juice of 1 lemon
¼ teaspoon ground cumin
Kosher salt
Freshly ground black pepper
3 avocados, cubed
1 pint cherry tomatoes, halved
1 small cucumber, sliced into
　 half moons
⅓ cup corn kernels
1 jalapeño, minced (optional)
2 tablespoons chopped cilantro

1. In a small bowl, whisk together oil, lemon juice, and cumin. Season dressing with salt and pepper.

2. In a large serving bowl, combine avocados, tomatoes, cucumber, corn, jalapeño (if using), and cilantro. Gently toss with dressing and serve immediately.

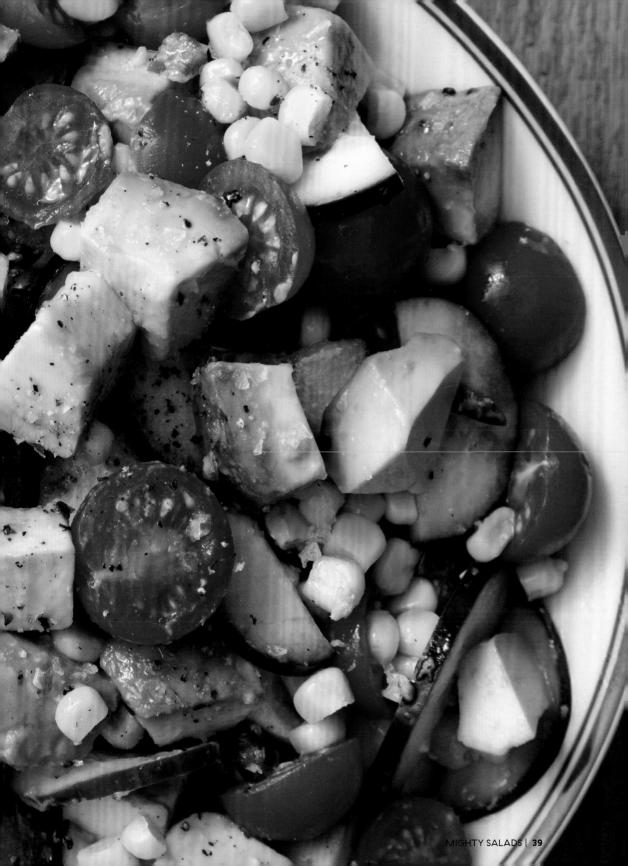

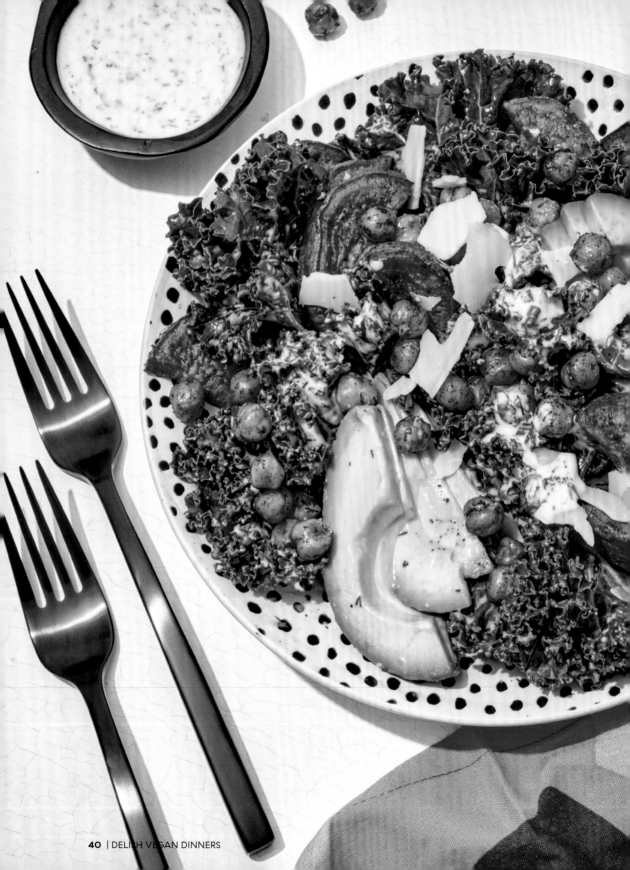

Coconut Kale Salad

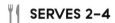 **SERVES 2-4** | **TOTAL TIME: 1 HR 10 MIN**

We love the subtle notes of coconut in this creamy dairy-free ranch dressing. Massaging the kale helps break down its fibers, making for a more tender bite.

FOR THE COCONUT RANCH

¼ cup canned coconut milk
¼ cup vegan mayonnaise
1 tablespoon freshly chopped parsley
1 tablespoon freshly chopped chives
2 teaspoons freshly chopped dill
½ teaspoon garlic powder
¼ teaspoon onion powder
Pinch of cayenne
Kosher salt
Freshly ground black pepper

FOR THE SALAD

1 large sweet potato, cut into ¼-inch-thick half moons
1 tablespoon plus 2 teaspoons extra-virgin olive oil, divided
1½ teaspoons chili powder, divided
Kosher salt
Freshly ground black pepper
1 (15-ounce) can chickpeas, drained and rinsed
1 large bunch curly kale, washed and dried, stems removed
Avocado, thinly sliced
Shaved vegan Parmesan

1. In a small bowl, whisk together coconut milk and mayonnaise. Add herbs, garlic powder, onion powder, and cayenne. Stir to combine, then season with salt and pepper. Refrigerate until ready to use.

2. Preheat oven to 400°F. Place sweet potatoes on a large baking sheet and drizzle with 1 tablespoon oil. Season with 1 teaspoon chili powder, salt, and pepper. Toss to coat, then spread potato slices in an even layer.

3. Bake until tender and bottoms start to crisp, 35 to 40 minutes.

4. Pat chickpeas dry with a paper towel and place on a small baking sheet. Bake until dried out and crisp, 30 minutes.

5. While chickpeas are still warm, place in a medium bowl. Add remaining 2 teaspoons oil and ½ teaspoon chili powder. Toss to combine and season with salt and pepper.

6. Roughly chop kale into bite-size pieces and transfer to a large bowl. Add a large pinch of salt and massage kale with your fingers, rubbing salt in for about 1 minute.

7. Top kale with sweet potatoes, chickpeas, avocado, and Parmesan. Drizzle with coconut ranch to serve.

Lentil Salad

This super-versatile lentil salad is a meal prepper's dream. It's healthy, it's flexible, it keeps for a full week, and it tastes better the longer it sits! Have we convinced you yet?

FOR THE SALAD

1 tablespoon extra-virgin olive oil
½ large yellow onion, diced
1 medium carrot, finely chopped
Kosher salt
Freshly ground black pepper
1 teaspoon chopped fresh thyme
½ teaspoon smoked paprika
2½ cups cooked green lentils
   (from about 1 cup dried)
½ cup freshly chopped herbs, such
   as basil, parsley, mint, or chives
¼ cup roasted chopped nuts, such
   as walnuts, pecans, almonds,
   cashews, or pistachios

FOR THE VINAIGRETTE

2 tablespoons extra-virgin olive oil
2 tablespoons white wine vinegar
½ shallot, minced
2 teaspoons Dijon mustard
1 teaspoon lemon zest
Kosher salt
Freshly ground pepper

1. In a large skillet over medium heat, heat oil. Add onion and carrot and season with salt and pepper. Cook, stirring occasionally, until onions are tender and translucent, about 6 minutes. Add thyme and paprika and cook until fragrant, 1 minute.

2. Turn off heat and make vinaigrette: Whisk together all vinaigrette ingredients and season to taste with salt and pepper.

3. Add lentils, herbs, nuts, and vinaigrette to skillet with carrots and onions. Stir to combine then let sit 10 minutes to allow lentils to absorb dressing. Transfer to serving bowl and serve immediately.

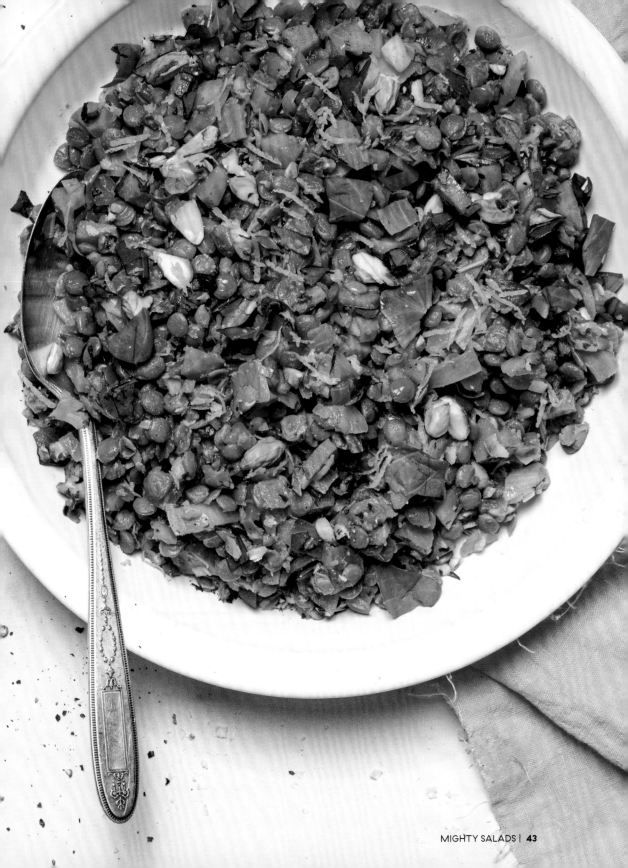

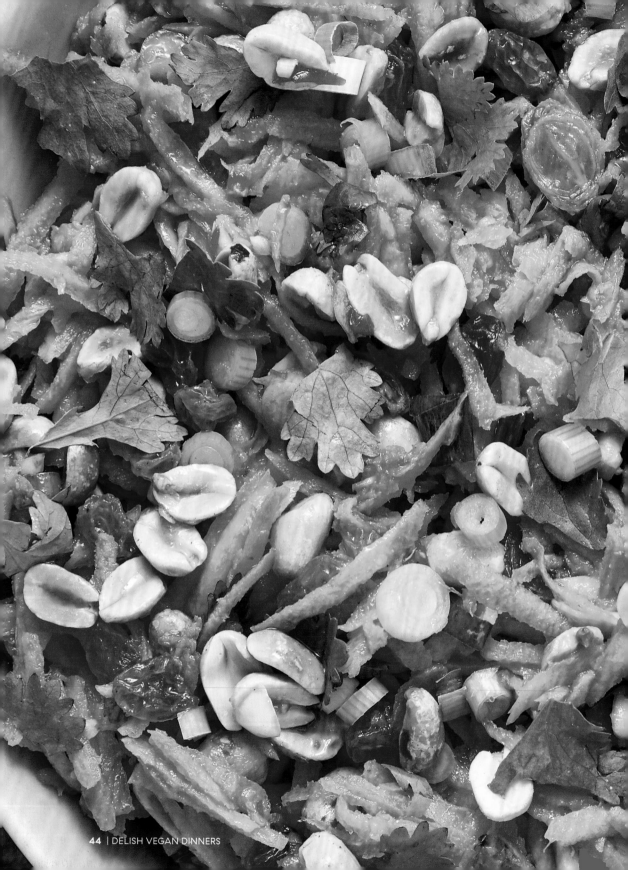

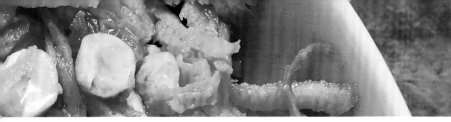

Moroccan Carrot Salad

 SERVES 6 | **TOTAL TIME: 25 MIN**

If you're not familiar with harissa, the fiery Tunisian chile paste, this salad is the perfect place to start. Sweet golden raisins and roasted peanuts offset the bright, assertive flavors in the dressing.

1 pound carrots, peeled and
   grated (about 3 cups)
¾ cup golden raisins
¾ cup toasted peanuts
¼ cup freshly chopped cilantro
2 green onions, thinly sliced
¼ cup extra-virgin olive oil
1 to 2 tablespoons harissa,
   depending on spice preference
1 tablespoon agave syrup
Juice and zest of 1 lime
2 cloves garlic, minced
2 teaspoons freshly grated ginger
1 teaspoon ground cumin
Kosher salt
Freshly ground black pepper

1. In a large bowl, toss together carrots, raisins, peanuts, cilantro, and green onions.

2. In a medium bowl, whisk together oil, harissa, agave, lime juice and zest, garlic, ginger, and cumin. Pour dressing over carrot mixture and toss to coat. Season with salt and pepper.

Classic Shallot Vinaigrette

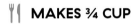 **MAKES ¾ CUP** | 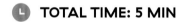 **TOTAL TIME: 5 MIN**

Keep this easy dressing in your back pocket and you'll never touch the bottled stuff again. Every vinegar is different, so adjust your olive oil according to taste. You're looking for a particular balance; aim to curb the vinegar's sharpness without allowing the rich flavor of the olive oil to dominate.

½ large shallot, minced (about
   3 tablespoons)
2 tablespoons vinegar (such
   as white wine, apple cider,
   champagne, or red wine)
2 teaspoons Dijon mustard
⅓ to ½ cup extra-virgin olive oil
Kosher salt
Freshly ground black pepper

1. In a medium bowl, whisk together shallot, vinegar, and mustard. Slowly stream in olive oil, whisking constantly, until mixture is smooth and emulsified. Season to taste with salt and freshly ground pepper.

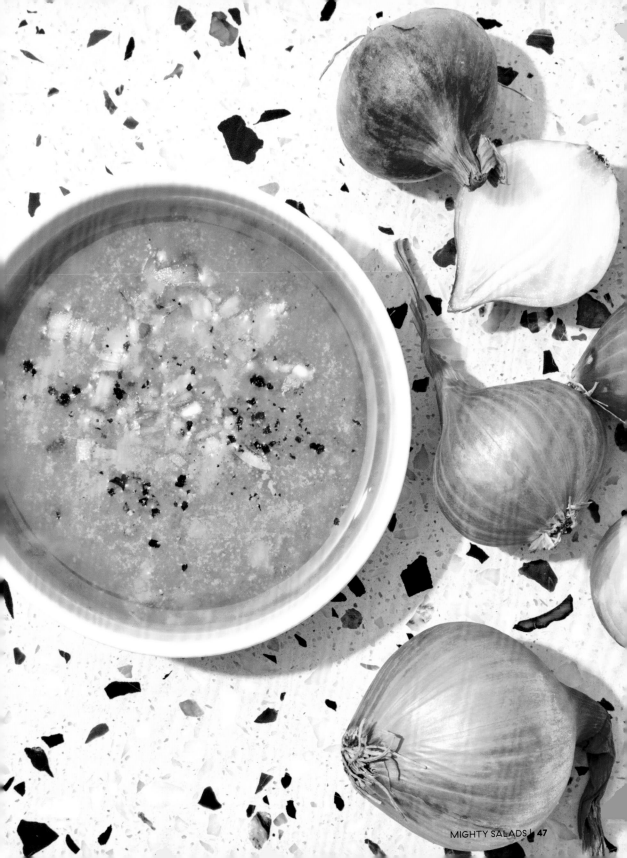

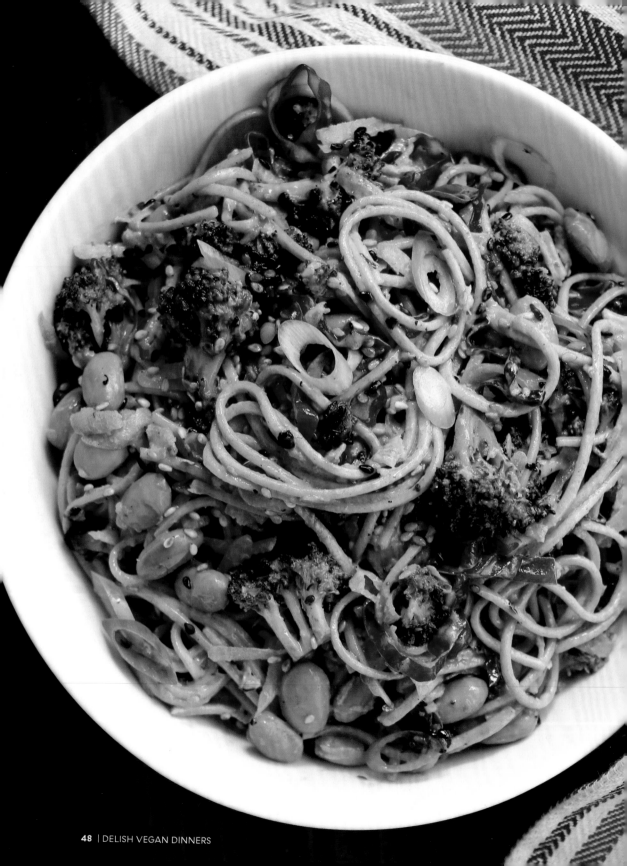

Creamy Noodle Salad

This flexible pasta salad is substantial enough to be a full-on meal. Sub in your favorite veggies and noodle, but don't skimp on the spicy mayo dressing.

FOR THE DRESSING

¼ cup vegan mayonnaise

2 tablespoons Sriracha

Zest of ½ lime (optional)

1 tablespoon rice wine vinegar

1½ teaspoons granulated sugar

1 clove garlic, grated

1-inch piece ginger, grated

½ teaspoon kosher salt

FOR THE SALAD

4 ounces soba noodles

4 teaspoons toasted sesame oil, divided

1 tablespoon extra-virgin olive oil

1 small head broccoli, cut into 1-inch florets (about 2 cups)

2 cloves garlic, minced

2 tablespoons hoisin sauce

Juice of ½ lime (optional)

1 tablespoon sesame seeds, plus more for garnish

2 medium carrots, grated (about 1¼ cups)

1 cup shredded red cabbage

¾ cup edamame, blanched

1 green onion, thinly sliced, for serving

2 tablespoons freshly chopped cilantro, for garnish (optional)

1. In a large bowl, whisk together all dressing ingredients until smooth.

2. In a large pot of salted boiling water, cook noodles according to package directions until just short of al dente (3 to 4 minutes if using soba noodles). Drain immediately. Add noodles and 1 teaspoon sesame oil to dressing bowl and toss to coat evenly. Set aside.

3. Cook broccoli: In a medium skillet over medium-high heat, heat olive oil. Add broccoli and cook, stirring occasionally, until broccoli is lightly charred, about 5 minutes. Stir in remaining 3 teaspoons sesame oil and garlic and cook until fragrant, 30 seconds. Remove from heat and toss with hoisin sauce, lime juice (if using), and sesame seeds until evenly coated.

4. To bowl with noodles, add carrots, cabbage, edamame, and broccoli and toss until well combined.

5. Garnish with green onions, cilantro (if using), and more sesame seeds before serving.

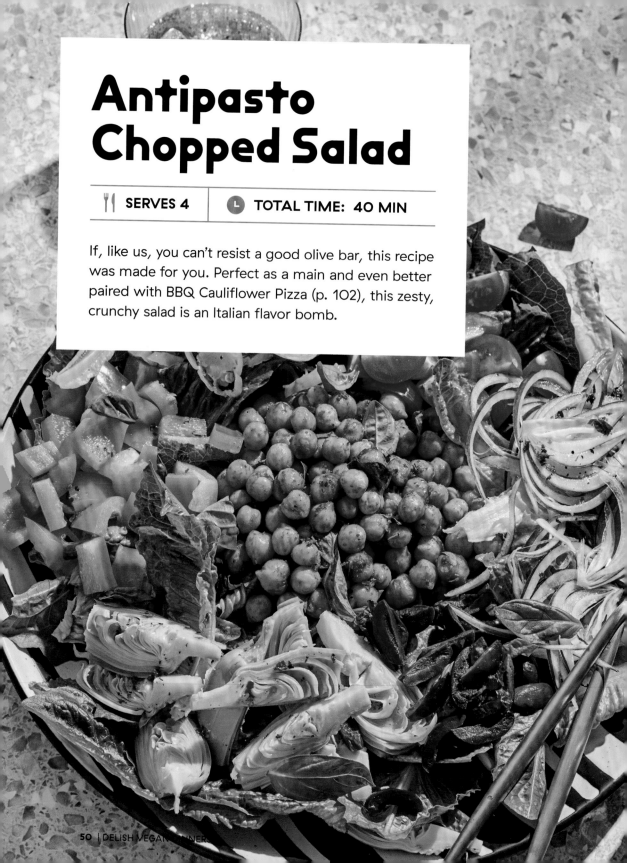

Antipasto Chopped Salad

¶¶ SERVES 4	🕐 TOTAL TIME: 40 MIN

If, like us, you can't resist a good olive bar, this recipe was made for you. Perfect as a main and even better paired with BBQ Cauliflower Pizza (p. 102), this zesty, crunchy salad is an Italian flavor bomb.

FOR THE DRESSING

⅓ cup extra-virgin olive oil

3 tablespoons white wine vinegar

1½ teaspoons Italian seasoning

1 small garlic clove, finely grated
   or minced

Pinch of red pepper flakes

Kosher salt

Freshly ground black pepper

FOR THE SALAD

1 (15.5-ounce) can chickpeas,
   drained and rinsed

2 tablespoons chopped fresh basil
   leaves, plus more leaves torn for
   serving

¾ teaspoon sweet paprika

Kosher salt

Freshly ground black pepper

1 large head romaine lettuce,
   chopped (9 ounces)

1 cup canned artichoke hearts,
   drained and cut into bite-size
   pieces

¾ cup cherry tomatoes, quartered

½ cup sliced Kalamata or black
   olives

¼ cup sliced pepperoncini
   peppers

½ small red onion, thinly sliced

½ orange bell pepper, seeded,
   stemmed, and diced (¾ cup)
   and dried, stems removed

Avocado, thinly sliced

Shaved vegan Parmesan

1. Make dressing: In a medium jar with a tight-fitting lid, combine dressing ingredients. Season with salt and pepper. Shake until well combined.

2. Make salad: In a medium bowl, toss chickpeas with basil and paprika; season with salt and pepper. Fill bottom of a large serving bowl with romaine lettuce. Pile paprika chickpeas in center of lettuce. Arrange artichoke, tomatoes, olives, pepperoncini, red onion, and bell pepper around chickpeas.

3. Shake dressing to ensure it is well combined and pour over top of salad. Garnish with torn basil leaves. Toss before serving.

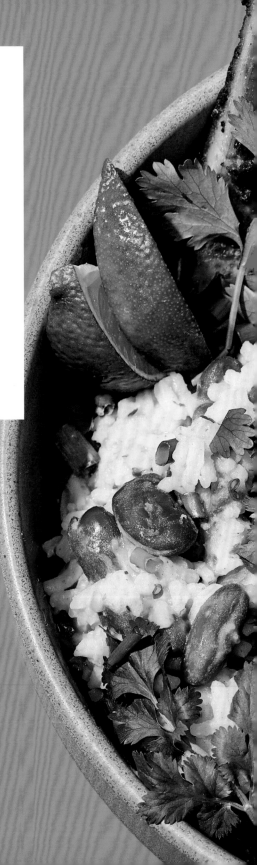

Have A Bowl Of Sunshine

This Jerk Tofu Grain Bowl has a little bit of everything: crunchy slaw, plantains, and flavor-packed tofu; all on a bed of coconut rice and peas.

TURN FOR THE RECIPE! $\longrightarrow$

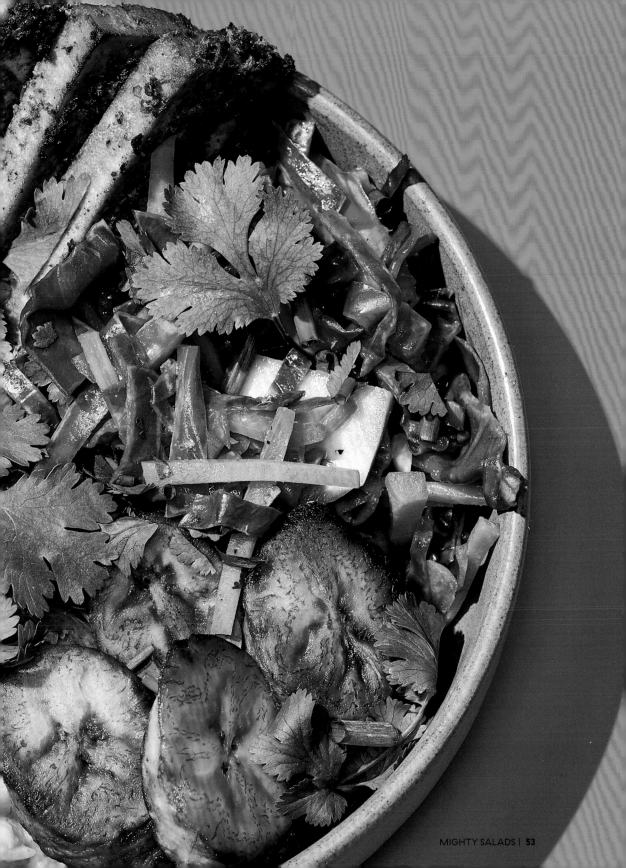

Jerk Tofu Grain Bowl

 SERVES 3–4 | **TOTAL TIME: 2 HR**

FOR THE FRIED PLANTAINS

Vegetable oil, for frying
2 large ripe plantains, sliced on
   a bias into ½-inch pieces
Kosher salt

FOR THE CABBAGE CARROT SLAW

1 small red cabbage, shredded
1 large carrot, thinly sliced into
   matchsticks
1 teaspoon kosher salt
2 tablespoons extra-virgin olive oil
2 tablespoons apple cider vinegar
Juice of 1 lime
½ tablespoon agave syrup
½ tablespoon Dijon mustard
Kosher salt
Freshly ground black pepper

FOR THE QUICK RICE & PEAS

1 (15-ounce) can red kidney
   beans, undrained
1 (7-ounce) can coconut milk
1 cup plus 2 tablespoons water
2 scallions, halved
10 allspice berries
3 cloves garlic
½ Scotch bonnet pepper, seeds
   removed
2 sprigs thyme
Kosher salt
Freshly ground black pepper
1 cup basmati rice

1. Fry plantains: Fill a large skillet with enough oil to just cover bottom of pan with oil. Heat over medium-high until oil shimmers. Carefully add plantain slices to pan in a single layer. Fry until plantains are a deep golden brown and can easily be pierced with a fork, 3 to 4 minutes a side. Remove to a paper towel–lined plate and season with salt.

2. Make slaw: In a large bowl, combine cabbage, carrots, and salt and set aside for 15 minutes. Squeeze cabbage mixture over sink to remove moisture

3. Meanwhile, in a small bowl, whisk olive oil, vinegar, lime juice, agave, and mustard until totally combined. Season with salt and pepper to taste. Toss cabbage with dressing to coat and chill.

4. Make rice and peas: In a medium saucepan over medium heat, add kidney beans, coconut milk, and water. Add scallions, allspice berries, garlic, Scotch bonnet, thyme, a generous pinch of salt and black pepper. Bring to a boil then reduce to a simmer and let cook uncovered for 20 minutes.

5. In a fine mesh strainer, rinse basmati under cold water until water runs clear. Remove scallions, allspice berries, and garlic. If a lot of liquid has evaporated, refill to original level with water, then bring to a boil. Add rice, reduce to a simmer, and cook covered for 15 to 20 minutes, or until rice is cooked through.

6. For tofu and bowls: In a food processor or blender, add onions, scallions, ginger, Scotch bonnets, thyme, 2 teaspoons allspice, soy sauce, and vinegar. Blend until a smooth paste has formed. Season with salt and pepper and set aside in a large bowl.

7. Slice tofu into ¼-inch slices and sprinkle both sides with remaining 1 teaspoon allspice, cinnamon, garlic

FOR THE TOFU & BOWLS

1 medium onion, roughly chopped

3 scallions, roughly chopped, plus more sliced for garnish

2-inch piece ginger, roughly chopped

2 Scotch bonnet peppers

3 sprigs thyme, leaves removed and stems discarded

3 teaspoons allspice, freshly ground if possible, divided

¼ cup low-sodium soy sauce

¼ cup apple cider vinegar

Kosher salt

Freshly ground black pepper

¼ teaspoon cinnamon

1 teaspoon garlic powder

2 (16-ounce) packages extra-firm tofu, drained and pressed

Extra-virgin olive oil

Cilantro, finely chopped, for garnish

Lime wedges

powder, salt, and pepper. Add tofu to jerk marinade and carefully toss to coat, making sure to not break slices. Cover with plastic wrap and chill for 2 hours or up to overnight.

8. Preheat oven to 400°F and arrange a rack in top and middle of oven. On a parchment-lined baking tray, lay tofu in a single layer, making sure some of marinade has adhered to the slices. Drizzle lightly with olive oil and roast on middle rack for 30 minutes, until edges have browned and jerk seasoning has darkened slightly. Move tray to top rack and broil on high for 2 to 3 minutes, or until tofu has begun to char in places.

9. To serve, layer rice, 3 to 4 slices of tofu, plantains, and slaw in a large bowl. Garnish with thinly sliced scallion, a sprinkle of cilantro, and lime wedges.

PRO TIP!

If Scotch bonnet peppers aren't available, go for habaneros instead.

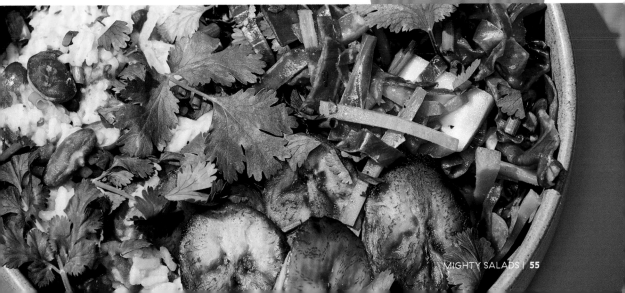

Super Green Pasta Salad

It's not so hard to eat your greens when they come in pasta salad form. Sweet baby spinach is great here, but peppery arugula or tender baby kale would work well too.

FOR THE SALAD

Kosher salt

8 ounces elbow macaroni

3 cups packed fresh spinach

1 cup frozen green peas or edamame, defrosted and drained

2 Persian cucumbers, quartered lengthwise and chopped

½ cup freshly chopped herbs, such as parsley, basil, or cilantro

2 jalapeños, thinly sliced into rounds

3 tablespoons capers, drained

2 teaspoons lemon zest

1 avocado, cubed

¼ cup toasted hulled pumpkin seeds

Freshly ground black pepper

Crushed red pepper flakes

FOR THE DRESSING

3 tablespoons lemon juice

½ medium shallot, minced

1 teaspoon agave syrup

⅓ cup extra-virgin olive oil

Kosher salt

Freshly ground black pepper

1. In a large pot of salted boiling water, cook pasta until al dente. Drain pasta in a colander then run under cold water to stop cooking and rinse off starches. Set aside to drain while you make dressing.

2. Make dressing: In a medium bowl, whisk together lemon juice, shallot, and agave. Whisking constantly, slowly drizzle in olive oil until mixture is emulsified. Season with salt and pepper.

3. In a large bowl, combine pasta, spinach, peas, cucumbers, herbs, jalapeños, capers, and lemon zest. Toss for 1 to 2 minutes, until spinach has reduced in volume and become slightly wilted. Add avocado and pumpkin seeds and toss gently until just combined. Season to taste with salt, pepper, and crushed red pepper flakes.

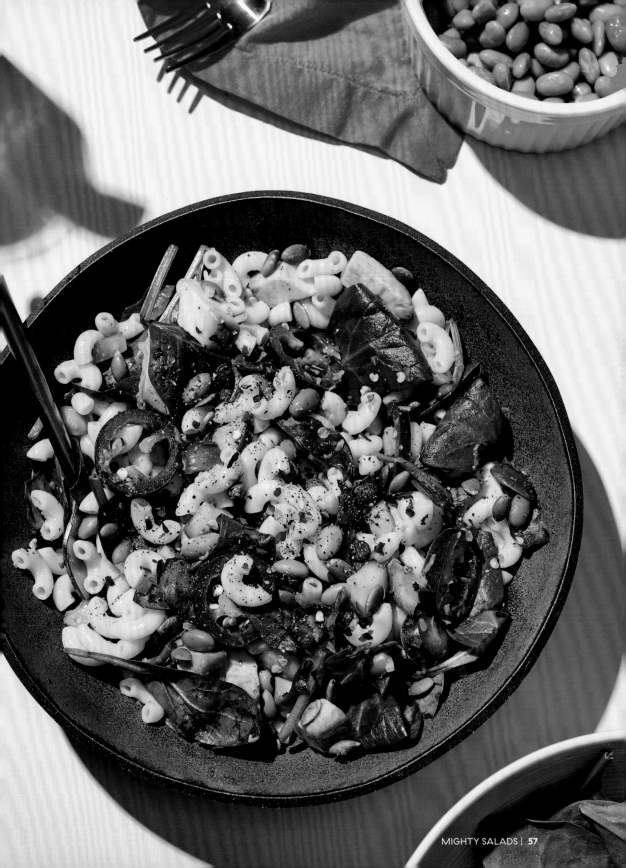

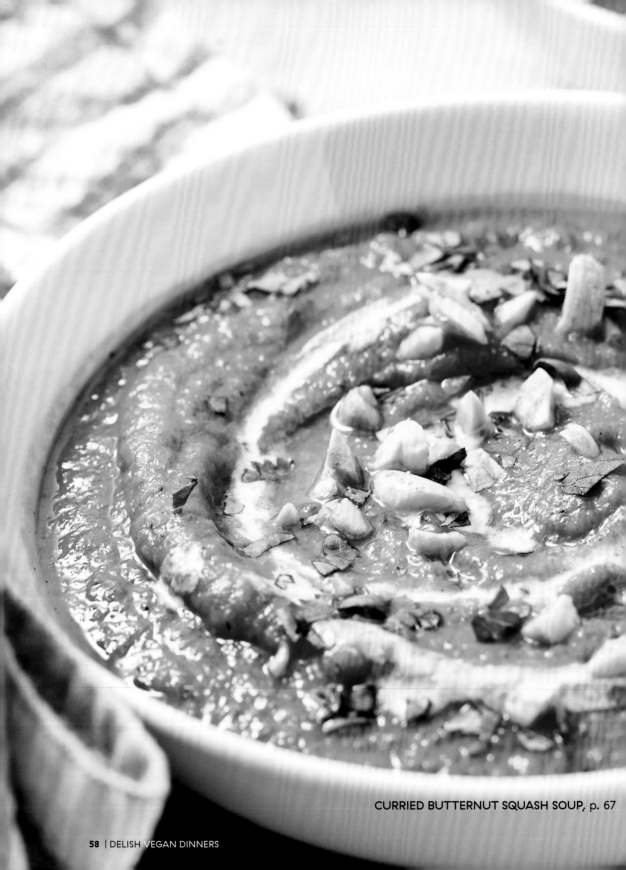

CURRIED BUTTERNUT SQUASH SOUP, p. 67

CHAPTER THREE

BEST-EVER SOUPS

Easy bowls that will comfort you again and again.

White Bean & Kale Soup

 SERVES 4 | **TOTAL TIME: 45 MIN**

Beans are the key to this (creamless!) creamy soup. Use the back of your wooden spoon to smash about a quarter of the beans into the side of your pot, then stir to combine. They'll essentially melt into the soup, creating a velvety, substantial broth.

1 tablespoon extra-virgin olive oil
½ yellow onion, finely chopped
2 stalks celery, finely chopped
1 leek, cleaned and thinly sliced
   (white and pale green parts only)
3 cloves garlic, minced
2 teaspoons freshly chopped
   thyme
½ teaspoon red pepper flakes
   (optional)
Kosher salt
Freshly ground black pepper
4 cups low-sodium vegetable
   broth
2 cups water
2 (15.5-ounce) cans cannellini
   beans, drained and rinsed
Juice of 1 lemon
1 large bunch lacinato kale,
   removed from stems and torn
   into medium pieces
Vegan Parmesan, for serving

1. In a large pot over medium heat, heat oil. Add onion, celery, and leek and cook until slightly soft, 6 minutes. Add garlic, thyme, and red pepper flakes (if using) and cook until fragrant, 1 minute. Season with salt and pepper.

2. Add broth, water, and beans and bring to a simmer. Stir occasionally, mashing some beans in pot to thicken soup. Let simmer 15 minutes then stir in lemon juice and kale. Cook until wilted, 3 minutes.

3. Garnish with vegan Parmesan before serving.

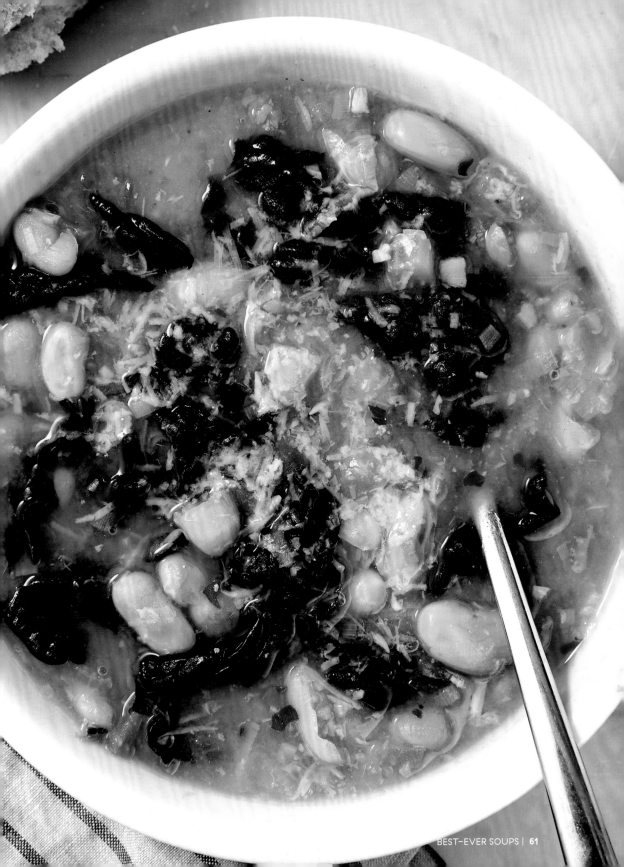

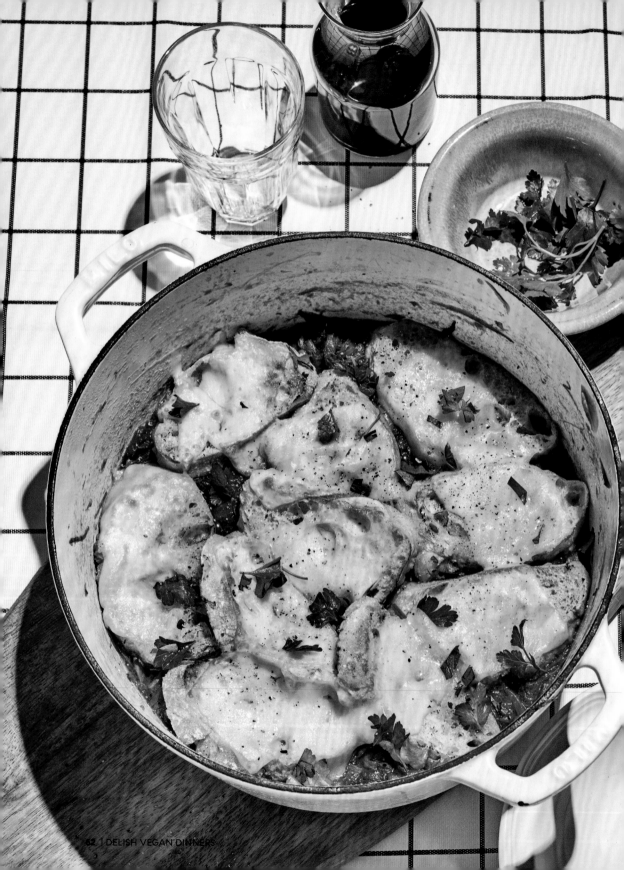

French Onion Lentil Stew

 SERVES 4–6   **TOTAL TIME: 1 HR 15 MIN**

Broiling the toasts right in the soup pot makes for an impressive presentation. But if you're meal prepping, it's best to do that job on a sheet tray instead; you'll avoid losing soggy pieces of bread in your leftovers.

---

5 cups water, divided
Extra-virgin olive oil
¾ pound (about 2 large) yellow onions, thinly sliced ¼ inch thick
¾ pound (about 4 small) red onions, thinly sliced
Kosher salt
Freshly ground black pepper
½ cup dry red wine
3 sprigs fresh thyme
4 cloves garlic, finely chopped
2 bay leaves
½ cup brown lentils
½ sliced baguette
Preferred sliced vegan cheese, such as provolone or Gruyère
Freshly chopped parsley, for serving

1. Fill a measuring cup with 1 cup cold water. In a large skillet over medium-high heat, heat 1 tablespoon olive oil. Add a large handful of sliced onions and season with salt and pepper. Cook, stirring occasionally, until onions are tender and browned, 8 to 10 minutes. Transfer cooked onions to a large oven-safe soup pot then return skillet to burner. Add a splash (about 2 tablespoons) of water from measuring cup to skillet to deglaze pan, using wooden spoon to scrape up any browned bits. Transfer liquid to soup pot with cooked onions and wipe skillet clean. Repeat process with remaining onions. (To expedite this process, multiple large skillets can be used to cook onions simultaneously.)

2. When all onions are cooked and in soup pot, add any remaining water from previously measured 1 cup, wine, thyme, garlic, and bay leaves to pot. Bring up to a simmer and cook for 5 minutes. Add remaining 4 cups water and lentils and bring up to a boil. Reduce heat to low and simmer, skimming foam from surface and stirring occasionally, until lentils are tender, 30 to 35 minutes.

3. When lentils are tender, remove pot from heat and preheat oven broiler to high. Top soup with baguette pieces, then top with cheese. Place pot in oven and broil until cheese is melty, 2 to 5 minutes depending on your broiler and cheese. Sprinkle with parsley before serving.

Tortilla Soup

 SERVES 4–6 | **TOTAL TIME: 1 HR 20 MIN**

Beware, this recipe has some kick! If it tastes a little too spicy at the end of cooking, add 1 to 2 tablespoons of brown sugar to mellow the heat. Or, if your goal is a milder soup, skip the jalapeño altogether.

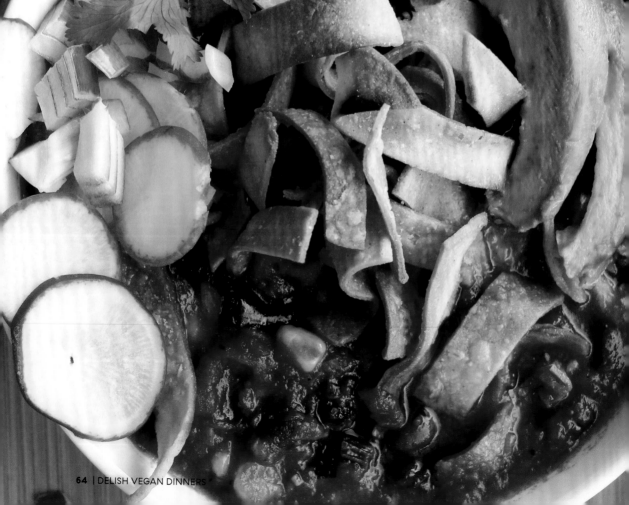

½ cup extra-virgin olive oil

8 small corn tortillas, halved and sliced into ½-inch-wide strips

Kosher salt

1 jalapeño, seeds removed and diced

1 poblano, seeds removed and diced

1½ teaspoons ground cumin

1 teaspoon ground coriander

1 teaspoon smoked paprika

½ teaspoon freshly ground black pepper

1 teaspoon kosher salt

1 large red onion, diced, divided

5 cloves garlic, minced

2 tablespoons tomato paste

2 chipotles in adobo, diced

1 (15-ounce) can hominy, drained

1 cup corn

1 (15.5-ounce) can black beans, drained and rinsed

1 (14.5-ounce) can fire-roasted diced tomatoes

1 (28-ounce) can crushed tomatoes

2 cups low-sodium vegetable broth or water

Fried tortilla chips

Sliced avocado

Sliced radishes (optional)

Diced red onion

Cilantro (optional)

Lime wedges

1. Make tortilla chips: In a small pot over medium heat, heat oil. Frying in 2 batches, add half the tortilla strips and fry until golden, stirring frequently, about 6 minutes. Transfer fried chips onto a paper towel–lined plate and immediately sprinkle with salt while hot. Repeat with remaining tortilla strips. Reserve oil.

2. Make soup: In a large pot over medium-high heat, heat 2 tablespoons reserved tortilla frying oil. Add jalapeño and poblano and let cook until slightly charred, stirring occasionally, about 8 minutes. Add cumin, coriander, paprika, pepper, and salt and stir until fragrant, about 1 minute.

3. Reserve ¼ cup of diced onion for topping. Add remaining onion and garlic to pot and let cook, stirring occasionally, until onions begin to turn golden, about 7 minutes. Add tomato paste and stir until color deepens, about 1 minute. Add chiles and adobo sauce and stir until evenly distributed and fragrant, 1 minute.

4. Add hominy, corn, beans, tomatoes, and broth. Bring to a simmer then reduce heat to low. Let cook for at least 20 minutes; for a thicker soup, let cook longer to desired consistency.

5. Top soup with crispy tortilla strips, avocado, radish, onion, cilantro, and a wedge of lime.

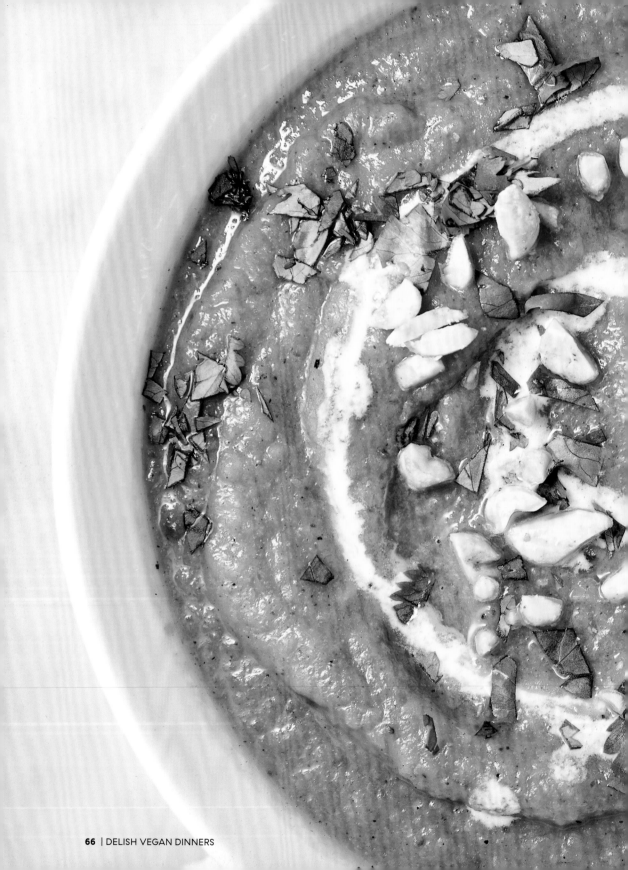

Curried Butternut Squash Soup

 SERVES 4–6   **TOTAL TIME: 1 HR**

A drizzle of creamy coconut milk along with a scattering of crunchy peanuts and bright cilantro make for a particularly beautiful bowl of this classic fall soup.

2 pounds butternut squash, peeled and chopped
3 tablespoons melted coconut oil
1 red onion, quartered
2 large carrots, roughly chopped
3 cloves garlic
Kosher salt
Freshly ground black pepper
2 tablespoons curry powder
4 cups low-sodium vegetable broth, warmed
½ cup canned coconut milk
¼ cup peanuts, roughly chopped
Freshly chopped cilantro, for garnish

1. Preheat oven to 425°. On 2 large, rimmed baking sheets, toss squash with oil, onion, carrots, and garlic. Season with salt, pepper, and curry powder.

2. Bake, tossing occasionally, until squash is caramelized and tender, about 45 minutes.

3. Add squash mixture to blender with broth and puree until creamy.

4. Drizzle coconut milk over each serving and garnish with peanuts and cilantro.

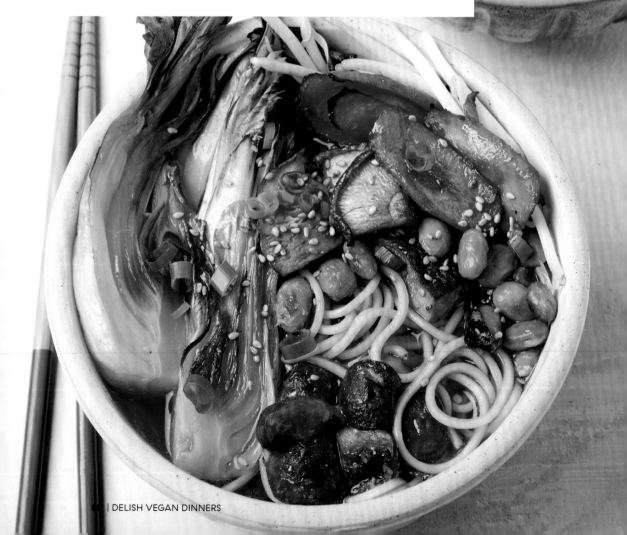

Red Miso Veggie Ramen

 SERVES 4 | **TOTAL TIME: 1 HR 5 MIN**

New to dried kombu? It's a variety of seaweed that will impart a rich, mushroom-like flavor to your broth. Don't fear the white powder on the outside: that's where much of the umami goodness lies.

FOR THE BROTH

2 tablespoons vegetable oil

1 medium yellow onion, chopped

1 large carrot, peeled and sliced

1 (4-inch) piece ginger, cut into
   ¼-inch slices

10 cloves garlic, peeled, smashed

Kosher salt

5 ounces fresh shiitake mushrooms,
   stems removed, caps reserved

2 (3-inch) segments kombu (the
   more dusty, white powder, the
   better!)

½ ounce dried shiitake mushrooms

2 heads baby bok choy, quartered

6 green onions, chopped

4 cups low-sodium vegetable
   broth

FOR THE VEGGIES

1 tablespoon red miso paste

2 tablespoons vegetable oil, divided

2 green onions, white parts minced,
   greens thinly sliced and reserved

1 teaspoon grated fresh ginger

2 cloves garlic, grated

1 large carrot, thinly sliced

5 ounces shiitake mushrooms
   (reserved caps only)

6 ounces baby portobello
   mushrooms, quartered, stems
   removed and discarded

2 heads baby bok choy, quartered

½ cup shelled edamame

Kosher salt

FOR SERVING

1 (10-ounce) pack dry ramen
   wheat noodles

¼ cup mirin

¼ cup low-sodium soy sauce

1 tablespoon toasted sesame seeds

Green onions

Sesame oil

1. Make broth: In a large Dutch oven, heat canola oil over medium heat. Add onion, carrot, ginger, garlic, and a heavy pinch of salt. Cook 7 minutes, stirring occasionally, or until veggies begin to take on some color.

2. Add shiitake stems, kombu, dried shiitake mushrooms, bok choy, and green onions. Add vegetable broth and 4 cups water. Bring to a boil over high heat then reduce to a simmer. Cover and cook for 25 minutes.

3. Strain broth through a fine-mesh strainer into a large clean bowl. With back of wooden spoon, press liquid out of stock veggies, mashing them with spoon. Discard strained vegetables.

4. Return broth to Dutch oven and season to taste with salt, keeping in mind soy sauce will be added later.

5. Make roasted vegetables: Preheat oven to 425°F. In a medium bowl, combine miso paste, 1 tablespoon oil, green onion, ginger, and garlic.

6. Toss carrots and mushrooms separately in miso mixture then transfer to a foil-lined, rimmed baking sheet, keeping each vegetable separate. Leave enough room to add bok choy and edamame. Roast for 5 minutes.

7. In a medium bowl, toss bok choy and edamame with oil and season with salt. Add bok choy and edamame to baking sheet and roast for another 15 minutes, or until all veggies are tender and golden.

8. In a large pot of salted boiling water, cook ramen noodles according to package instructions then drain.

9. In a small bowl, whisk together mirin and soy sauce.

10. Add 1½ cups hot broth to each bowl. Divide noodles among bowls then top each with carrots, mushrooms, and bok choy. Drizzle each bowl with soy-mirin mixture then garnish with roasted edamame, green onions, sesame oil, and sesame seeds before serving.

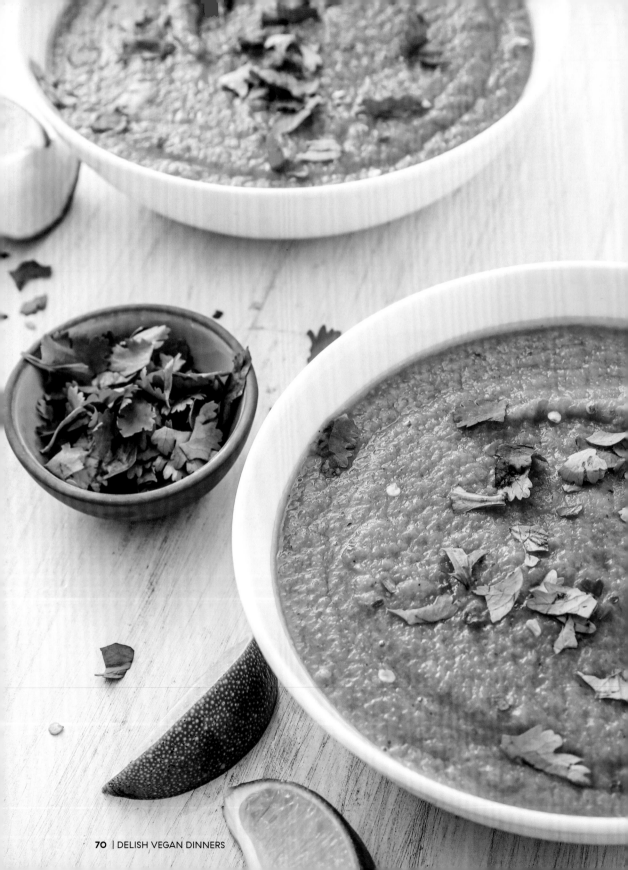

Carrot & Coriander Soup

 MAKES 6 | **TOTAL TIME: 1 HR 15 MIN**

Our secret for a perfectly balanced carrot soup? Start by roasting—not boiling—your carrots. A trip to a hot oven will deepen their earthy sweetness.

2 pounds carrots, peeled and cut into 2-inch pieces
4 tablespoons extra-virgin olive oil, divided
1 teaspoon ground coriander
Kosher salt
Freshly ground black pepper
1 large red onion, chopped
2 cloves garlic, minced
1 jalapeño, seeds removed and finely chopped
¼ cup packed fresh cilantro leaves plus stems, separated, plus more leaves for garnish
6 cups low-sodium vegetable broth
Pinch of crushed red pepper flakes
Lime wedges, for serving

1. Preheat oven to 425°. Toss carrots with 2 tablespoons oil, coriander, salt, and pepper on a large baking sheet. Roast until carrots are fork-tender, 30 minutes.

2. In a large pot over medium heat, heat remaining 2 tablespoons oil. Add red onion and cook until soft, about 5 minutes.

3. Add garlic, jalapeño, and cilantro stems. Cook until fragrant, 1 minute more.

4. Add broth, cilantro leaves, red pepper flakes, and roasted carrots. Bring to a boil then reduce heat and let simmer 15 minutes.

5. Using a blender or an immersion blender, blend until smooth. If using a blender, carefully remove lid every so often to let steam escape.

6. Garnish with more cilantro and serve with lime wedges.

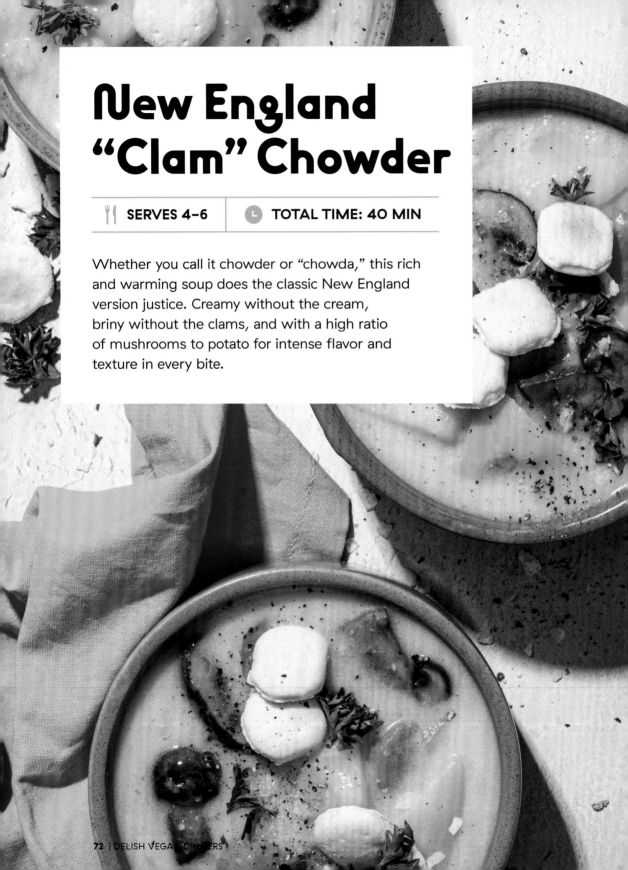

New England "Clam" Chowder

SERVES 4–6 | **TOTAL TIME: 40 MIN**

Whether you call it chowder or "chowda," this rich and warming soup does the classic New England version justice. Creamy without the cream, briny without the clams, and with a high ratio of mushrooms to potato for intense flavor and texture in every bite.

FOR THE SOUP

¼ cup vegan butter, divided
1 tablespoon extra-virgin olive oil
1 pound cremini mushrooms
Kosher salt
1 medium yellow onion, chopped
2 medium carrots, trimmed and
   thinly sliced into rounds
4 cloves garlic, minced
1 tablespoon miso
½ cup white wine
2 cups water
1 bay leaf
2 pounds Yukon gold potatoes,
   peeled and chopped (roughly
   ¾-inch cubes)
Freshly ground black pepper
Chopped fresh curly parsley
   leaves, for serving
oyster crackers, for serving

FOR THE "CREAM" SAUCE

2 large russet potatoes, peeled
and chopped
2 cups unsweetened almond milk

1. Make soup: Place a medium pot over medium-high heat. Add 2 tablespoons butter, oil, and mushrooms; season with salt. Cook, stirring occasionally, until any liquid mushrooms release cooks off and they are tender but still chewy like clams, about 5 minutes. Remove mushrooms to a plate.

2. Return pot to medium heat. Add remaining 2 tablespoons of butter, onion, and carrot and cook, stirring occasionally, until onions are softened, about 3 minutes.

3. Add garlic to pot and cook, stirring, 2 minutes, until garlic is lightly toasted. Stir in miso.

4. Add wine and increase heat to medium-high. Bring to a boil and cook until wine evaporates, about 3 minutes.

5. Pour water into pot and add Yukon gold potatoes. There should be just enough water to cover potatoes. Season with salt and bring to a boil. Cover pot, reduce heat to medium, and simmer until potatoes and carrots are tender, about 10 minutes.

6. Meanwhile, make "cream" sauce: In a small saucepan, cover russet potatoes with at least 1 inch of water. Place over medium-high heat and bring to a boil. Reduce heat to medium and cook until potatoes are very tender, about 7 minutes. Drain.

7. Scrape cooked potatoes into a blender carafe and add almond milk. Blend until a smooth puree forms. Set aside until ready to use.

8. Finish soup: When vegetables are tender, remove lid from pot and pour in "cream." Stir to fully combine. Season with salt and pepper.

9. Right before serving, stir cooked mushrooms back into pot and ladle soup into bowls. Top each bowl with parsley and oyster crackers.

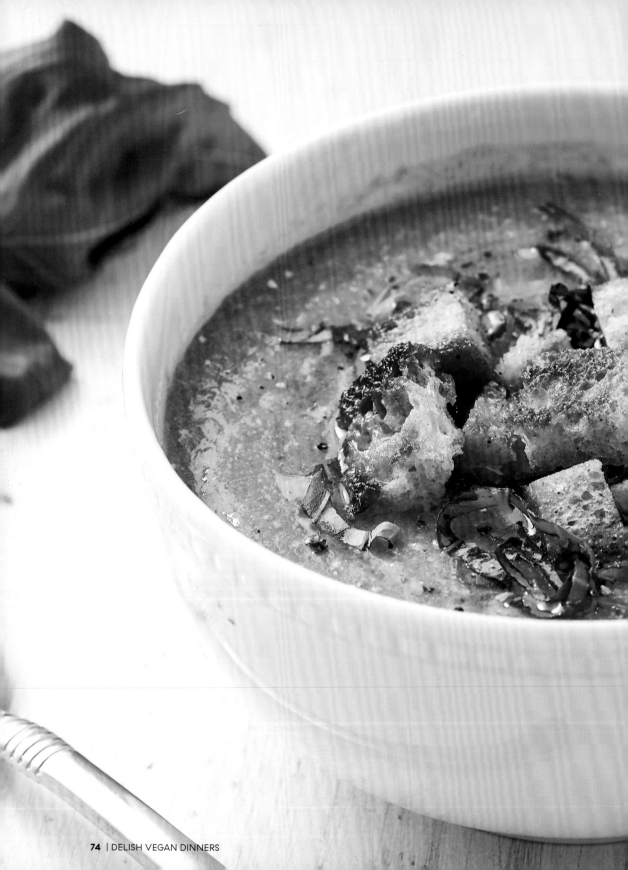

Gazpacho

 SERVES 3 | **TOTAL TIME: 25 MIN**

The better the tomato, the better the gazpacho, meaning you're gonna want to save this recipe for the heat of summer (unless you live somewhere where ripe tomatoes are available year round). Acidity and sweetness vary depending on the tomato, so you may want to use more or less vinegar to perfectly balance the flavors.

2 pounds tomatoes, quartered

2 Persian cucumbers, peeled and chopped

½ red bell pepper, chopped

1 clove garlic, roughly chopped

2 tablespoons red wine or sherry vinegar

½ cup water

⅓ cup extra-virgin olive oil, plus more for garnish

Kosher salt

Freshly ground black pepper

2 slices country bread, cubed

2 tablespoons thinly sliced basil

1. Combine tomatoes, cucumbers, bell pepper, garlic, vinegar, and water in bowl of food processor or blender. Blend until smooth then add olive oil and blend to combine. Taste and season with salt, pepper, and more vinegar if needed. Cover and refrigerate until chilled.

2. Meanwhile, in a large skillet over medium heat, add enough olive oil to coat bottom of pan. Add cubed bread and cook, stirring occasionally, until bread is golden and crisp. Remove from heat, season with salt, and let cool.

3. To serve, divide soup among bowls and top with basil, croutons, and a drizzle of olive oil.

Chickpea Noodle Soup

Whether you're hungover, heartbroken, or just plain hangry, you can count on this homey soup to make it all a little better. Cooking the pasta in the soup will create a luxurious broth. (For a leftover–friendly version, boil the noodles separately so they don't bloat in the broth.)

2 tablespoons extra-virgin olive oil

½ medium yellow onion, chopped

1 shallot, chopped

2 stalks celery, chopped

2 medium carrots, cut into ¼-inch rounds

Kosher salt

Freshly ground black pepper

3 cloves garlic, minced

1 (15-ounce) can chickpeas, drained and rinsed

2 bay leaves

2 sprigs fresh rosemary

4 cups low-sodium vegetable broth

2 cups cold water

2 (2-inch-long) strips lemon peel

6 ounces orecchiette

3 tablespoons white miso paste

Crushed red pepper flakes

Freshly chopped dill, for garnish

Lemon wedges, for serving

1. In a large pot over medium heat, heat oil. Add onion and shallot and cook, stirring occasionally, until both have softened, 5 to 6 minutes. Add celery and carrots, season with salt and pepper, and cook for 5 minutes.

2. Add garlic and cook until fragrant, 1 minute. Add chickpeas, bay leaves, and rosemary and stir to combine. Season with salt and pepper and cook, stirring frequently, until you can smell rosemary, about 1 minute.

3. Add broth, water, and lemon peel and stir, scraping up any browned bits from bottom of pan. Bring up to a simmer, add pasta, bring mixture back up to a simmer, and cook, stirring occasionally, until pasta is cooked al dente, 13 to 15 minutes.

4. Remove soup from heat. Add miso to a medium bowl then ladle in about ½ cup broth from soup. Whisk until miso has totally dissolved into broth then stir mixture into soup. Season to taste with salt, pepper, and red pepper flakes. Ladle soup into bowls, garnish with dill, and serve with lemon wedges.

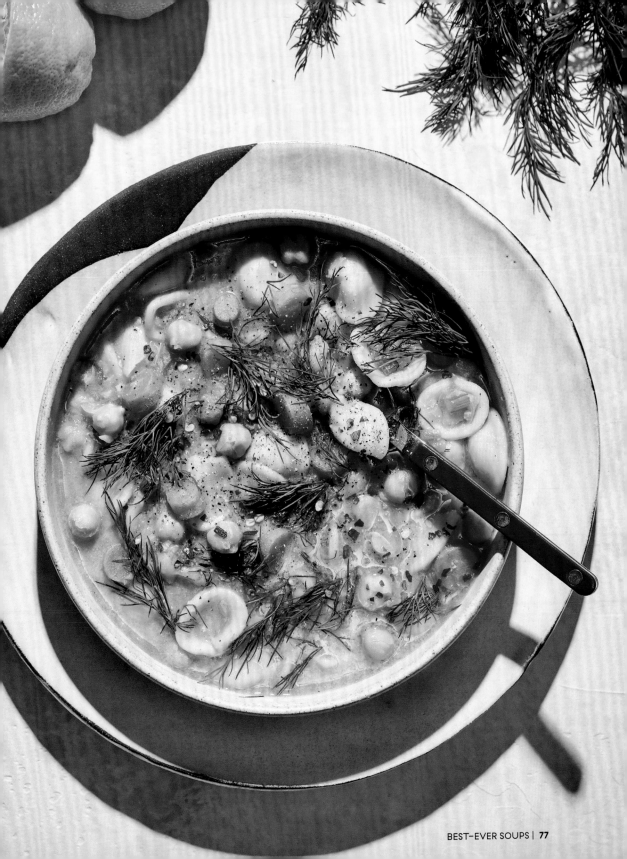

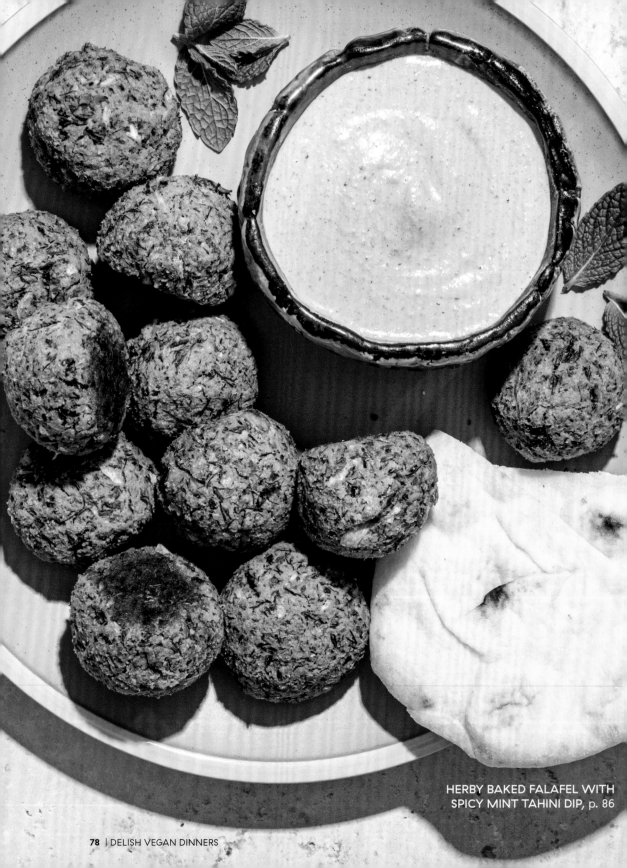

HERBY BAKED FALAFEL WITH
SPICY MINT TAHINI DIP, p. 86

CHAPTER FOUR

EASY WEEKNIGHTS

Short on time doesn't have to
mean short on flavor.

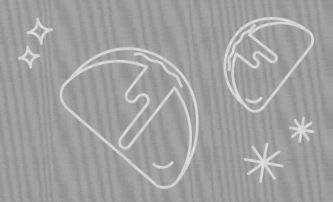

Chipotle Lentil Tacos

 SERVES 3-4 | **TOTAL TIME: 40 MIN**

Smoky spiced lentils make for an especially satisfying taco filling, and a creamy garlic–spiked avocado sauce cuts through the heat.

FOR THE SAUCE

½ ripe avocado
Juice of 1 lime
1 tablespoon extra-virgin olive oil
¼ cup fresh cilantro leaves and
   tender stems
1 garlic clove, minced
½ teaspoon kosher salt
⅔ cup cold water

FOR THE LENTIL FILLING

1 tablespoon extra-virgin olive oil
½ yellow onion, finely chopped
2 garlic cloves, minced
3 tablespoons tomato paste
1 chipotle pepper in adobo sauce
1 teaspoon ground cumin
½ teaspoon ground coriander
Kosher salt
2½ cups cooked green lentils
   (from about 1 cup dried)
¼ cup cold water

FOR SERVING

8 corn tortillas, warmed
Pickled red onions
Cilantro leaves, for serving
Thinly sliced Fresno chile

1. Make creamy avocado sauce: Combine all ingredients in a blender or food processor. Blend until smooth.

2. Make lentil filling: In a large skillet over medium heat, heat oil. Add onion and cook until soft, 6 minutes. Add garlic and cook until fragrant, 1 minute more.

3. Add tomato paste and chipotle pepper, and cook, mashing pepper with a wooden spoon, until tomato paste has darkened slightly, 2 minutes. Add cumin and coriander and season with salt.

4. Add lentils and cold water. Stir to combine, then cook, stirring and mashing some lentils occasionally, until lentils are heated through and partially mashed and no liquid remains, about 5 minutes. Add more water a tablespoon at a time if skillet becomes dry.

5. Assemble tacos: Fill each tortilla with a big spoonful of lentil mixture, a drizzle of sauce, red onions, cilantro, and Fresno chile.

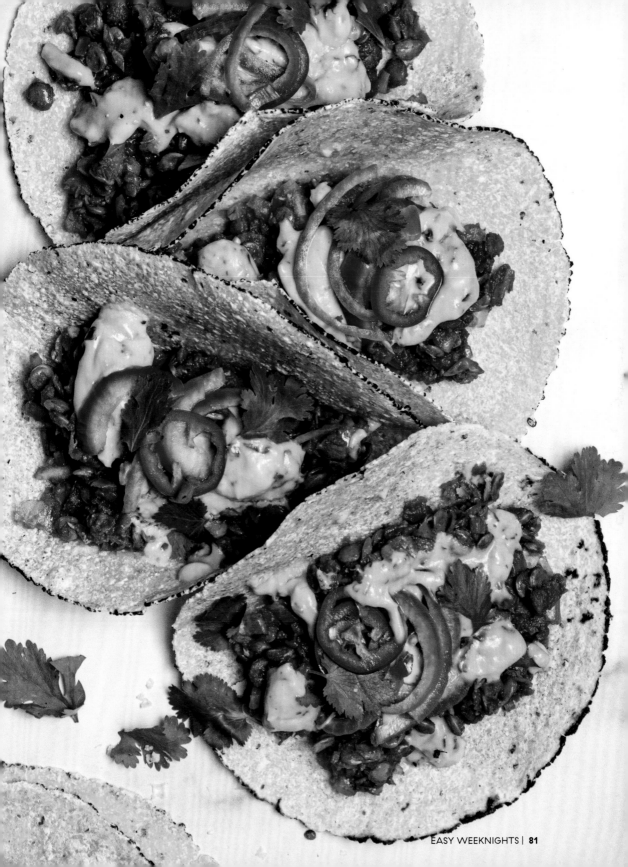

Tofu Bánh Mì

🍴 SERVES 4	🕐 TOTAL TIME: 40 MIN

In this meat-free Vietnamese classic, the pressed tofu will marinate twice: once quickly before cooking so it doesn't soak up too much liquid and again longer after it's cooked, to flavor it throughout. A French baguette will do the job, but getting your hands on an airier, lighter, thin-and-crisp-crusted Vietnamese baguette is the ultimate.

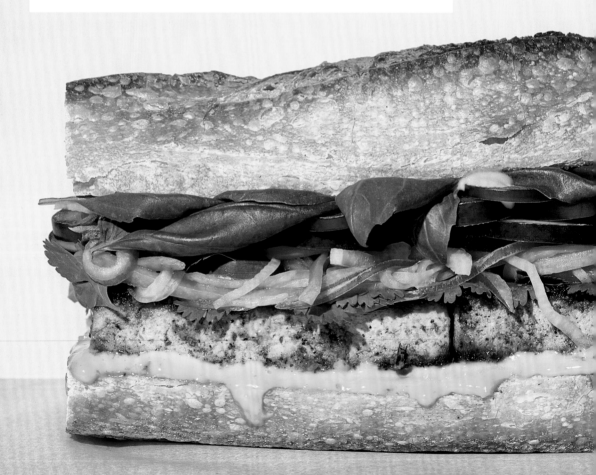

1 (14-ounce) block extra-firm tofu, drained and sliced into 8 equal slabs

FOR THE PICKLED VEGETABLES

1 small carrot, julienned (about 1 cup)

1 small daikon, julienned (about 1 cup)

½ small red onion, thinly sliced (about ½ cup)

1 cup unseasoned rice wine vinegar

3 tablespoons maple syrup

2 teaspoons kosher salt

FOR THE SPICY MAYO

¼ cup vegan mayonnaise

1 tablespoon Sriracha

FOR THE MARINADE

¼ cup low-sodium soy sauce

2 tablespoons sesame oil

2 tablespoons maple syrup

3 cloves garlic, peeled

3-inch piece lemongrass, roughly chopped

½-inch piece fresh ginger

⅓ cup cilantro, leaves and tender stems, roughly chopped

¾ teaspoon kosher salt

½ teaspoon freshly ground black pepper

FOR THE SANDWICHES

2 tablespoons vegetable oil

1 baguette, halved lengthwise and cut into 4 equal portions

2 cups cilantro, tough ends removed

1 cup basil leaves

1 small cucumber, thinly sliced

2 jalapeños, seeds removed and thinly sliced

1. Dry the tofu: Line a baking sheet with a clean kitchen towel folded in half. Lay tofu slices in a single layer. Cover with another clean kitchen towel and baking sheet. Place a heavy pot on top to press out as much liquid as possible.

2. Make pickled vegetables: In a medium bowl, combine carrot, daikon, red onion, rice wine vinegar, maple syrup, and salt. Stir until salt is dissolved, then press vegetables down to submerge in pickling liquid as much as possible.

3. In a small bowl, combine mayo and Sriracha.

4. Make marinade: In a blender or using an immersion blender, blend soy sauce, sesame oil, maple syrup, garlic, lemongrass, ginger, cilantro, salt, and black pepper until smooth.

5. Transfer dried tofu to a large plate. Pour marinade all over to coat. Marinate up to 2 minutes so tofu does not soak up too much liquid.

6. In a large skillet over medium heat, heat oil. Gently shake marinade off tofu. Do not discard marinade. Cook tofu until browned, about 3 minutes per side. The tofu will release from pan when it's ready, so don't force it. Transfer tofu back into marinade for at least 10 minutes.

7. To assemble: Spread baguettes with spicy mayo. Layer with tofu. Add cilantro, basil, pickled vegetables (shaking off pickling liquid first), cucumber, and jalapeños.

Seitan "Lomo" Saltado

 SERVES 3–4   **TOTAL TIME: 30 MIN**

Some days, you just *need* fries for dinner. This Chinese–Peruvian dish (usually made with beef) is the perfect excuse to curb your spud craving.

2 tablespoons vegetable oil, plus more if needed

1 pound seitan, cut in strips

1 medium red onion, sliced

2 aji amarillo or Fresno chiles, seeded and sliced

2 Roma tomatoes, cored and sliced

3 cloves garlic, minced

Kosher salt

Freshly ground black pepper

¼ cup low-sodium soy sauce

3 tablespoons apple cider vinegar

½ (28-ounce bag) frozen french fries, prepared according to package instructions

2 tablespoons chopped cilantro, for garnish

1. In a large skillet over high heat, heat oil until it just starts to smoke. Add seitan and sear, stirring occasionally, for 4 to 5 minutes, or until it begins to caramelize.

2. If there is no visible oil in pan, add about a tablespoon more before adding red onion and aji amarillo. Cook, tossing constantly, for 3 minutes, or until onions have just started to soften. Add tomatoes and cook for 2 to 3 minutes, tossing them with ingredients in pan. Make sure tomatoes have not cooked down fully and still retain a bit of bite. Add garlic, season with salt and pepper, and let cook for another minute.

3. Reduce heat to medium and add soy sauce and vinegar, stirring until seitan and veggies are fully coated with sauce. Let sauce reduce for 1 to 1½ minutes, or until it has thickened slightly.

4. Remove skillet from heat and add fries, tossing until they have been fully incorporated. Garnish with cilantro and serve.

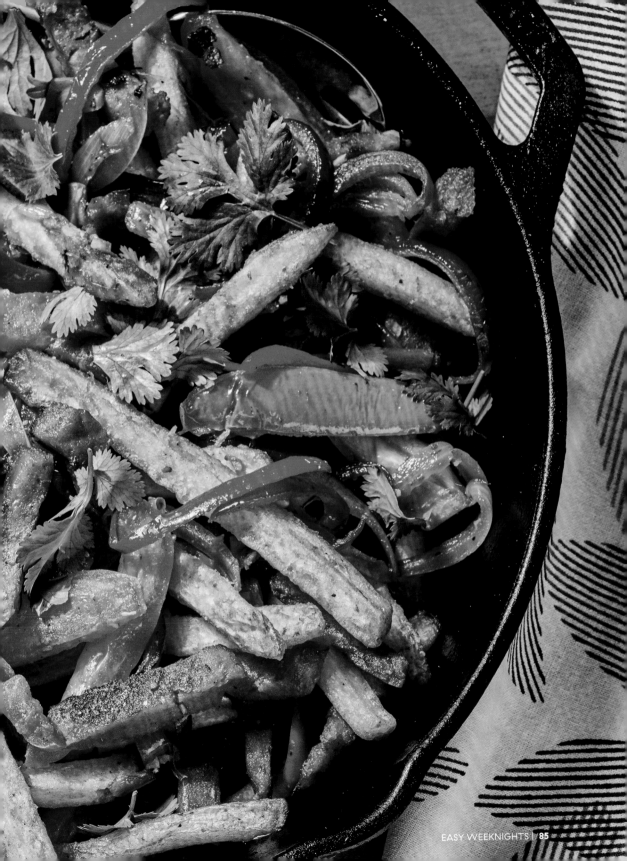

Herby Baked Falafel with Spicy Mint Tahini Dip

 SERVES 4 | 🕐 **TOTAL TIME: 35 MIN** |

Crispy on the outside and tender in the center, these baked falafel come together fast. They're delicious as is, or you can stuff them into pita with some fresh veggies for a more substantial meal.

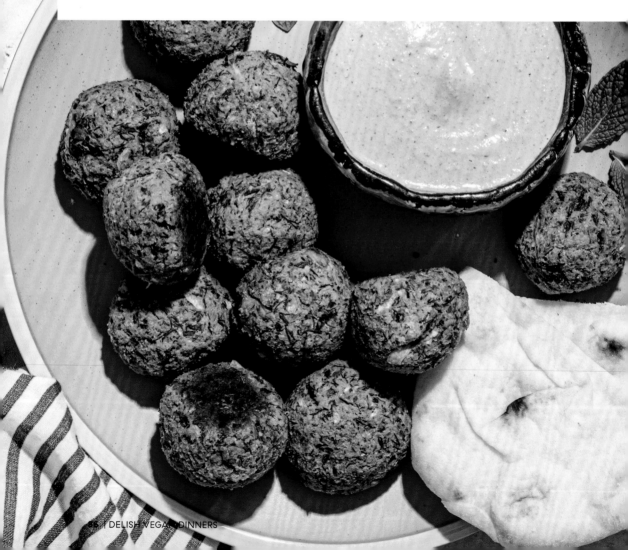

FOR THE FALAFEL

1 cup shelled pistachios

½ cup mint leaves

½ cup each cilantro, dill, and parsley (leaves and stems okay)

2 cups chickpeas, cooked or canned

2 cloves garlic

½ small yellow onion, chopped

3 tablespoons extra-virgin olive oil

1 tablespoon lemon zest, from 1 large lemon

1 tablespoon chickpea or all-purpose flour

1 teaspoon baking soda

1 teaspoon kosher salt

½ teaspoon ground coriander

½ teaspoon ground cumin

FOR THE SAUCE

½ cup tahini

½ cup mint leaves

2 tablespoons fresh lemon juice

1 teaspoon maple syrup

1 clove garlic

1 small jalapeño, seeds removed

½ teaspoon kosher salt

3 to 4 tablespoons water

1. Preheat oven to 425°F and line a baking sheet with parchment paper.

2. In a food processor, pulse nuts, mint, cilantro, dill, and parsley to finely chop. Add remaining ingredients and blend until you have a rough mash, scraping sides with a rubber spatula as you go.

3. Using your hands, form mixture into 20 balls and evenly space on prepared baking sheet. Bake 15 to 18 minutes, until lightly browned on bottoms.

4. Meanwhile, add all sauce ingredients, except water, to a blender. Blend, adding water 1 tablespoon at a time until smooth. Serve falafel with tahini sauce on the side.

PRO TIP!

A simple salad with chopped veggies dressed in the mint tahini sauce and topped with falafel makes a delicious lunch or dinner.

Chickpea "Tuna" Salad

  SERVES 4 | **TOTAL TIME: 5 MIN**

This quick "tuna" salad is proof that the magic is in the fixin's.
We always keep a can of chickpeas on hand so we're only ever
a few minutes away from this satisfying lunch.

1½ cups chickpeas (from 15-ounce
   can), rinsed and drained

3 tablespoons vegan mayonnaise

1 tablespoon Dijon mustard

1 stalk celery, finely chopped

¼ small red onion, finely chopped

1 tablespoon freshly chopped dill

Kosher salt

Freshly ground black pepper

Sliced whole wheat bread

Sliced tomatoes

Butter lettuce

Dill or bread and butter pickles

1. In a medium bowl, use a fork or potato masher to mash chickpeas into irregular-size pieces. (A few left whole is okay!)

2. Add mayonnaise, mustard, celery, onion, and dill and stir to combine. Season with salt and pepper to taste.

3. Assemble sandwiches on wheat bread topped with tomatoes, lettuce, and pickles.

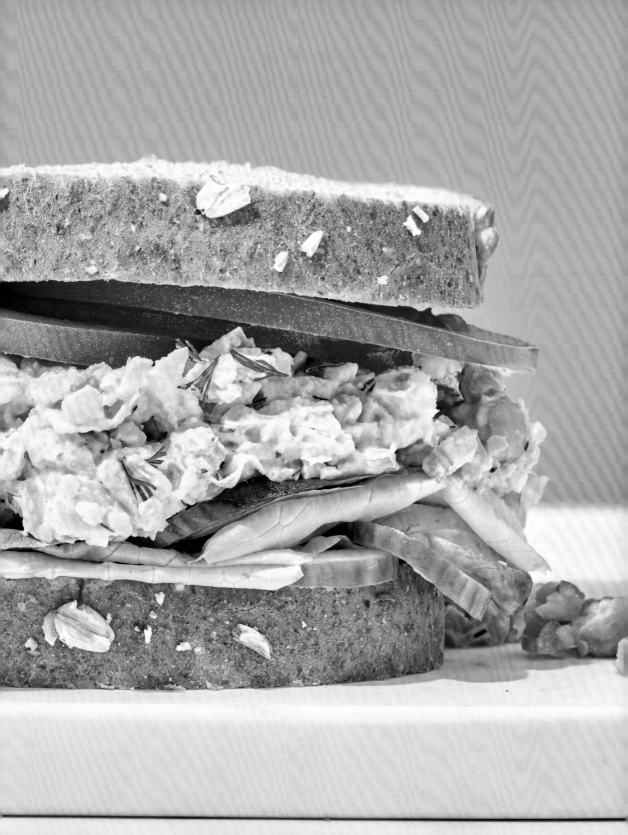

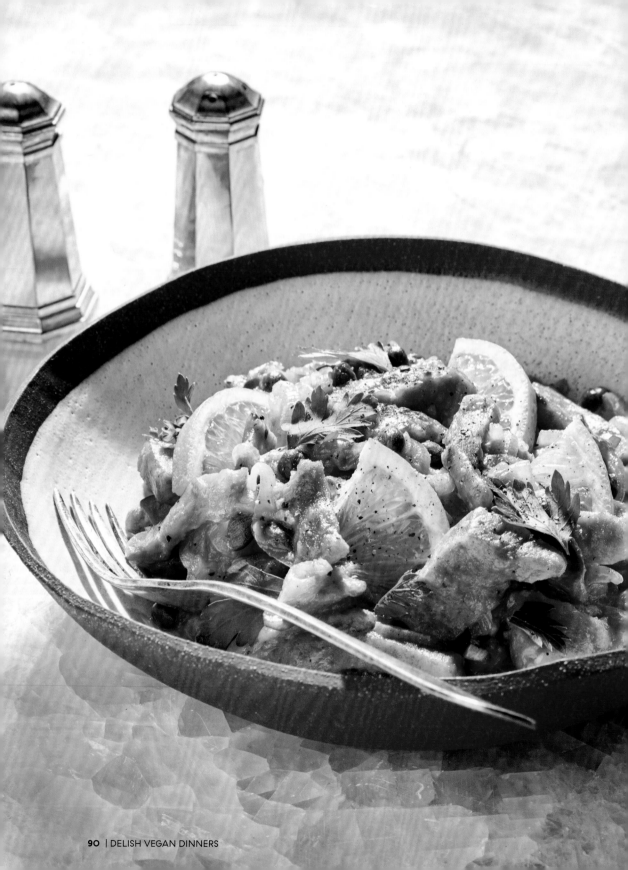

Extra Lemony Seitan Piccata

 SERVES 2 | **TOTAL TIME: 25 MIN**

Most piccata sauces use only lemon juice; we opt for whole pieces of the fruit to make use of every last bit of its bright citrus flavor. After a simmer in a wine and broth jacuzzi, the lemon loses its sharp bitterness, becoming sweet and tender. This piccata is great spooned over pasta or mashed potatoes, or accompanied by plenty of crusty bread.

1 (8-ounce) package seitan, torn into 2-inch pieces, or sliced into ¼-inch slices

Kosher salt

Freshly ground black pepper

1 tablespoon all-purpose flour

2 tablespoons vegan butter or extra-virgin olive oil, divided

1 medium shallot, halved and thinly sliced

2 garlic cloves, minced

¼ cup dry white wine

1½ cups low-sodium vegetable broth, divided

3 sprigs fresh thyme (optional)

½ lemon, washed, cut into thin rounds, seeded, and quartered

2 tablespoons capers, drained

Freshly chopped parsley, for serving

1. Place seitan pieces in a large bowl and season with salt and pepper. Add flour and toss until seitan is completely coated in flour.

2. Heat 1 tablespoon butter or oil in a large skillet over medium heat. Add seitan and cook, stirring or flipping occasionally, until golden brown on most sides, 4 to 5 minutes. (It's okay if some dry flour remains on seitan.) Transfer pieces to a plate and return skillet to medium heat.

3. Add another tablespoon of butter or oil then add shallot and garlic. Cook until fragrant, 1 minute, then add wine, using your spoon to scrape up any brown bits from bottom of pan. Add 1 cup broth and thyme, if using, and simmer for 5 minutes.

4. Stir in lemon pieces, capers, seared seitan, and remaining ½ cup vegetable broth and simmer 2 to 3 minutes more, until sauce has thickened to consistency of thin gravy. Season to taste with salt and pepper, garnish with parsley, and serve.

Tempeh & Broccoli Rabe Orecchiette

 SERVES 6 | **TOTAL TIME: 40 MIN**

Who needs a fancy Italian restaurant when you can make this 10-ingredient wonder in under an hour? Hearty tempeh stands in for the usual sausage, soaking up all that garlicky, lemony goodness. Broccoli rabe is classic, but broccoli florets will also do the trick.

1 pound broccoli rabe, ends trimmed

12 ounces orecchiette

3 tablespoons extra-virgin olive oil, plus more for serving

8 ounces tempeh, cut into ½-inch pieces

3 cloves garlic, minced

Kosher salt

Freshly ground black pepper

Red pepper flakes

Juice of ½ lemon

Vegan Parmesan, for serving

1. In a large pot of boiling salted water, blanch broccoli rabe for 3 minutes, or until it is bright green and tender. Transfer to a colander to drain, pressing on it with paper towel to help release excess water. Transfer to a cutting board and chop into bite-size pieces.

2. Return water to a boil and cook pasta until al dente according to package instructions. Reserve 1 cup of pasta water, then drain.

3. In a large skillet over medium heat, heat oil. Add tempeh and cook until golden and crispy, 6 to 8 minutes. Toward the end, when it is all mostly golden, break it up with a wooden spoon to create some smaller pieces. Remove from skillet and set aside to keep warm.

4. Return skillet to medium heat, adding more oil if necessary. Add garlic and cook until fragrant, 1 minute. Add broccoli rabe and cook 1 minute more. Season with salt, pepper, and a large pinch of red pepper flakes. Add pasta along with ½ cup reserved pasta water and lemon juice, tossing to combine. Return cooked tempeh to skillet and cook until warmed through. Add more pasta water as needed to thin out sauce and coat pasta. Season with salt and pepper to taste.

5. Serve with Parmesan and a drizzle of oil.

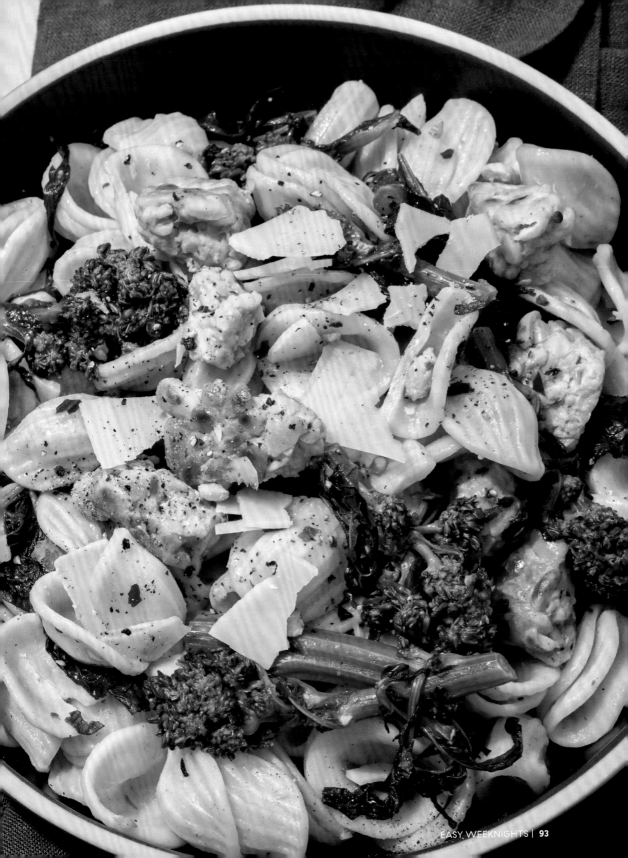

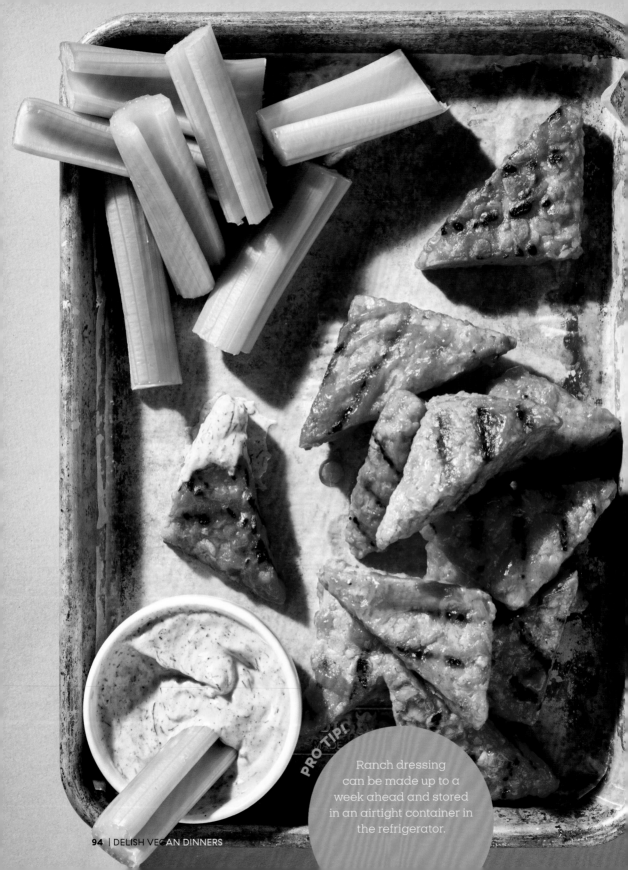

PRO TIP!

Ranch dressing can be made up to a week ahead and stored in an airtight container in the refrigerator.

Tempeh Buffalo "Wings"

 SERVES 4 | **TOTAL TIME: 35 MIN**

Quicker to make and easier to eat, these plant–based buffalo "wings" swap chicken for snackable triangles of tempeh. For a crowd, double or triple the recipe, steaming the tempeh in a large pot and working in batches on the grill.

FOR THE VEGAN RANCH

½ cup vegan mayonnaise
2 tablespoons fresh chopped dill
  fronds
1 tablespoon unsweetened
  almond milk, plus more if needed
1 tablespoon apple cider vinegar
¼ teaspoon garlic powder
¼ teaspoon onion powder
Large pinch of sweet paprika
Kosher salt
Freshly ground black pepper

FOR THE TEMPEH "WINGS"

2 (8-ounce) blocks tempeh
2 tablespoons safflower or
  vegetable oil, plus more for grill
½ cup hot sauce (such as Frank's)
½ cup vegan butter
1 tablespoon light agave syrup
4 celery stalks, cut into sticks,
  for serving

1. Make vegan ranch: In a medium bowl, whisk all ingredients until well combined. If mixture is too thick, stir in a little more almond milk or water. Season with salt and pepper.

2. Make tempeh "wings": Cut each block of tempeh crosswise into 3 pieces, then diagonally to create 6 triangular pieces per block. Fill bottom of a medium saucepan with 2 inches of water. Place saucepan over medium-high heat and bring to a simmer. Arrange tempeh pieces in an even layer in a steamer basket. Set basket in saucepan and cover. Reduce heat to medium and steam tempeh for 15 minutes.

3. Using tongs, remove pieces of tempeh to a medium bowl and toss with oil.

4. In a small saucepan, combine hot sauce, vegan butter, and agave syrup. Bring to a simmer and cook, whisking occasionally, until slightly reduced, about 6 minutes. Pour into a large heatproof bowl; keep warm.

5. Preheat grill or a grill pan to medium-high and oil grates. Add steamed tempeh and cook, turning occasionally, until golden on both sides, about 6 minutes. Transfer to bowl with buffalo sauce and toss well to coat. Serve with celery and ranch for dipping.

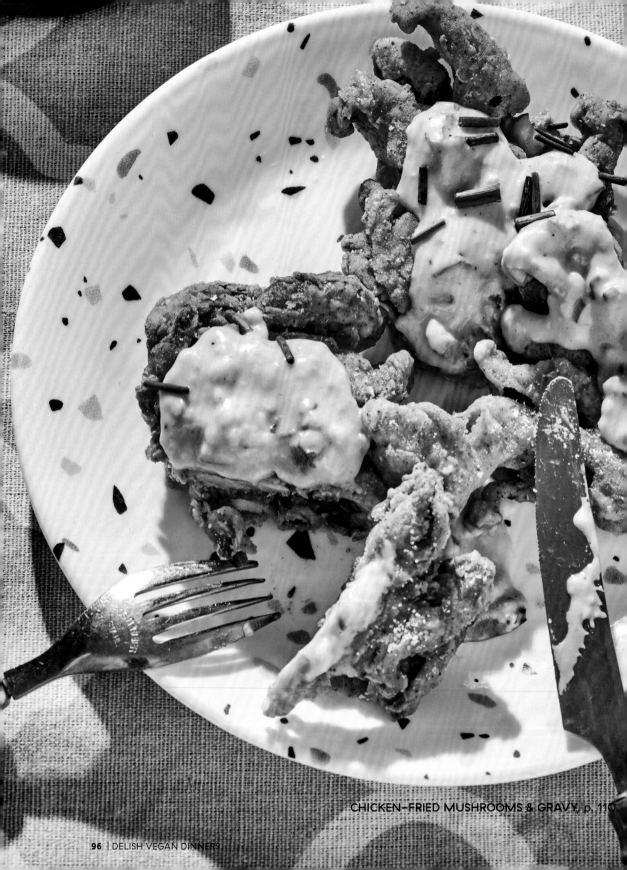

CHICKEN-FRIED MUSHROOMS & GRAVY, p. 110

CHAPTER FIVE

COMFORT FOOD

Satisfy your cravings for all things creamy, carby, and cozy.

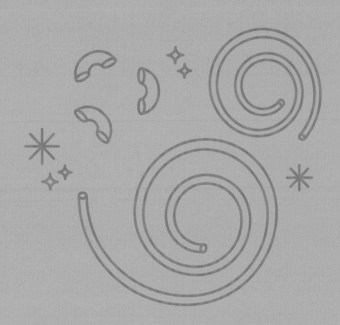

Creamy Mac & "Cheese"

 SERVES 6   🕐 **TOTAL TIME: 50 MIN**

Funky, briny sauerkraut and nutty nutritional yeast work together to create a seriously convincing sauce. The toasty, thyme–scented breadcrumb topping is just icing on the cake.

FOR THE PANKO TOPPING

2 tablespoons extra-virgin olive oil
½ cup panko bread crumbs
2 teaspoons fresh thyme leaves
Kosher salt
Freshly ground black pepper

FOR THE MAC & "CHEESE"

1 pound medium shells
1 tablespoon refined coconut oil
  or vegetable oil
1 white onion, chopped (about
  1½ cups)
½ medium yellow bell pepper,
  chopped (about 1 cup)
1 teaspoon ground mustard
1 teaspoon ground cumin
1½ cups raw cashews
1 russet potato, peeled and cubed
  (about 2 cups)
3½ cups water
⅔ cup sauerkraut, drained
3 tablespoons nutritional yeast
1 tablespoon white wine vinegar
1 tablespoon hot sauce (such as
  Cholula)

1. In a large pot of salted water, boil pasta until al dente, 9 to 10 minutes. Drain.

2. Meanwhile, make panko topping: In a medium skillet over medium heat, heat olive oil. Add panko, thyme and season with salt and pepper. Cook, stirring occasionally, until panko is golden. Transfer to a bowl to cool.

3. In a large pot over medium heat, heat coconut or vegetable oil. Add onion and bell pepper and cook until soft, 6 minutes. Season with salt and pepper, then stir in mustard and cumin and cook until fragrant, 1 to 2 minutes more. Add cashews, potatoes, and water and bring to a boil. Boil until potatoes are tender, 6 to 7 minutes.

4. When potatoes are tender, transfer mixture in pot to a blender or food processor; puree until smooth. Add sauerkraut, nutritional yeast, white wine vinegar, and hot sauce. Puree again until smooth then taste and season with salt and pepper, if needed.

5. In a large bowl, combine cooked pasta shells and "cheese" sauce and stir to combine. Top with panko mixture before serving.

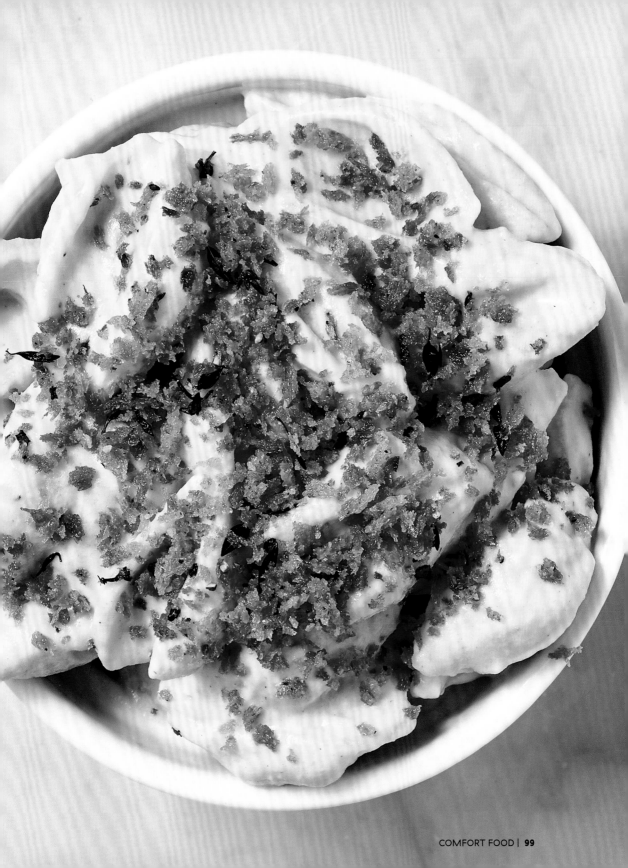

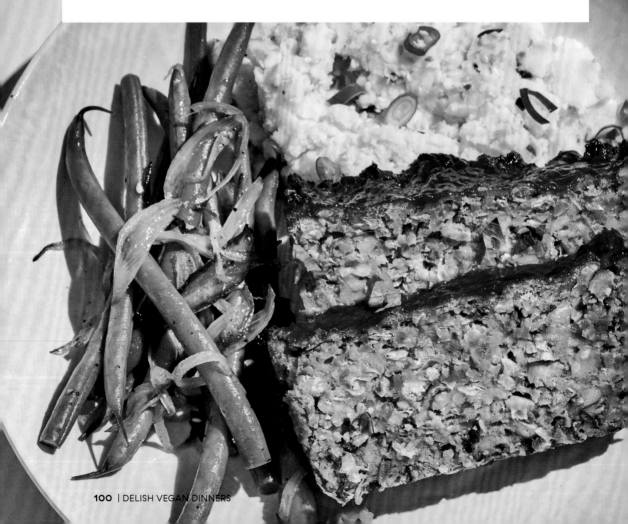

"Meatloaf" & Sesame Mashed Potatoes

 SERVES 8 | 🕐 **TOTAL TIME: 2 HR**

Loaded with hearty vegetables and umami–rich ingredients, this is not your grandmother's meatloaf. We love it served TV dinner–style, with mashed potatoes and crisp–tender steamed green beans. (P.S.: The leftovers make for a seriously good cold "meatloaf" sandwich. Thank us later.)

FOR THE "MEATLOAF"

1 tablespoon extra-virgin olive oil

½ yellow onion, finely chopped

2 stalks celery, finely chopped

1 medium carrot, peeled and finely chopped

1 cup finely chopped baby bella mushrooms

2 (15-ounce) cans chickpeas, drained and rinsed

1 cup panko bread crumbs

¼ cup freshly chopped parsley, plus more for garnish

2 tablespoons low-sodium soy sauce

1 tablespoon vegan Worcestershire sauce

¼ cup ketchup

¼ cup barbecue sauce

½ teaspoon smoked paprika

Kosher salt

Freshly ground black pepper

1. Preheat oven to 375°F and line an 5x8-inch loaf pan with parchment paper. In a large skillet over medium heat, heat oil. Add onion, celery, carrot, and mushrooms and cook, stirring occasionally, until vegetables are soft and most of the liquid has cooked out, 6 to 8 minutes.

2. Using a potato masher in a large bowl or food processor, mash the chickpeas until a rough paste forms. (A few large pieces of chickpea are okay.) Transfer to a large bowl if using a food processor.

3. Add cooked vegetables, bread crumbs, parsley, soy sauce, and Worcestershire sauce to bowl with chickpeas. In a medium bowl, whisk together ketchup and barbecue sauce. Add half of this mixture to bowl with chickpeas. Season with paprika, salt, and pepper and stir until all ingredients are evenly incorporated.

4. Transfer chickpea mixture to prepared loaf pan, packing in gently. Smooth top, then brush with half of remaining ketchup mixture and bake for 30 minutes. Remove from oven, brush with remaining ketchup mixture, and bake 30 minutes more.

5. Let cool 10 minutes, garnish with parsley, and serve.

FOR THE MASHED POTATOES

2 pounds Yukon gold potatoes, peeled and quartered

Kosher salt

3 tablespoons melted vegan butter

2 tablespoons toasted sesame oil

4 green onions, thinly sliced

2 cloves garlic, minced

Freshly ground black pepper

Toasted sesame seeds, for garnish

1. In a large pot, place potatoes and enough water to cover by at least 2 inches. Season well with salt. Bring to a boil and boil until potatoes are easily pierced with a fork, about 12 minutes. Drain and return potatoes to pot.

2. Mash potatoes with a wooden spoon or potato masher until they are almost smooth but big chunks remain. Add melted butter and oil and stir until well combined. Add most of green onions, saving some for garnish, and garlic and continue stirring until potatoes are desired consistency. Season with salt and pepper to taste.

3. Garnish with reserved green onions and toasted sesame seeds.

BBQ Cauliflower Pizza

 SERVES 2-4 | **TOTAL TIME: 1 HR**

Inspired by a *certain* pizza kitchen's iconic pie, this saucy, veggie-loaded number doesn't disappoint. Don't sleep on the vegan ranch; its creaminess is the perfect foil for the sweet and spicy barbecue-spiked cauli.

FOR THE PIZZA

½ small head cauliflower, cut into small florets
½ tablespoon extra-virgin olive oil
½ tablespoon apple cider vinegar
¼ teaspoon garlic powder
¼ teaspoon cayenne pepper
Kosher salt
Freshly ground black pepper
½ cup plus 2 tablespoons barbecue sauce, divided
Cooking spray, for pan
2 (8-ounce) packages store-bought pizza dough
¼ small red onion, thinly sliced

FOR THE VEGAN RANCH

½ cup vegan mayonnaise
Juice of 1 lemon
1 tablespoon finely chopped chives, plus more for garnish
1 tablespoon finely chopped parsley
1 clove garlic, minced
Kosher salt
Freshly ground black pepper

1. Preheat oven to 400°F. In a large bowl, toss cauliflower with oil, vinegar, garlic powder, and cayenne. Season with salt and pepper and spread in an even layer on a large baking sheet. Roast until florets are tender and slightly golden, 20 to 30 minutes, depending on floret size.

2. Return cauliflower to large bowl and toss with 2 tablespoons barbecue sauce. Turn oven up to 475°F. Grease 2 large baking sheets with cooking spray.

3. Make vegan ranch: In a medium bowl, mix together all ingredients then season with salt and pepper.

4. Flatten pizza dough into a large round on a prepared baking sheet. Spread ¼ cup barbecue sauce on crust in a thin, even layer, leaving about a ½-inch border. Top with half of the cauliflower and red onions. Repeat with second ball of dough, then bake both until crust is crispy, 12 to 15 minutes.

5. Garnish with chives and a drizzle of the vegan ranch.

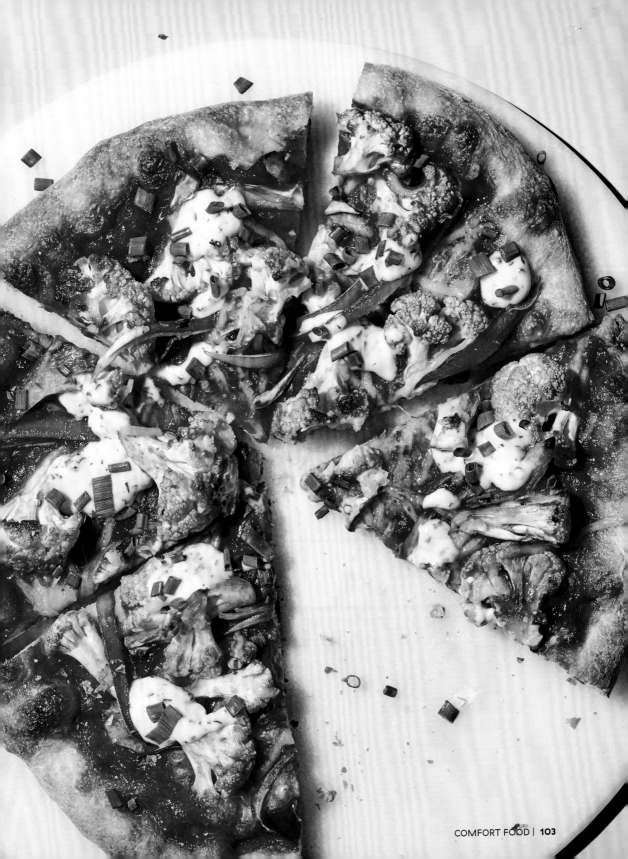

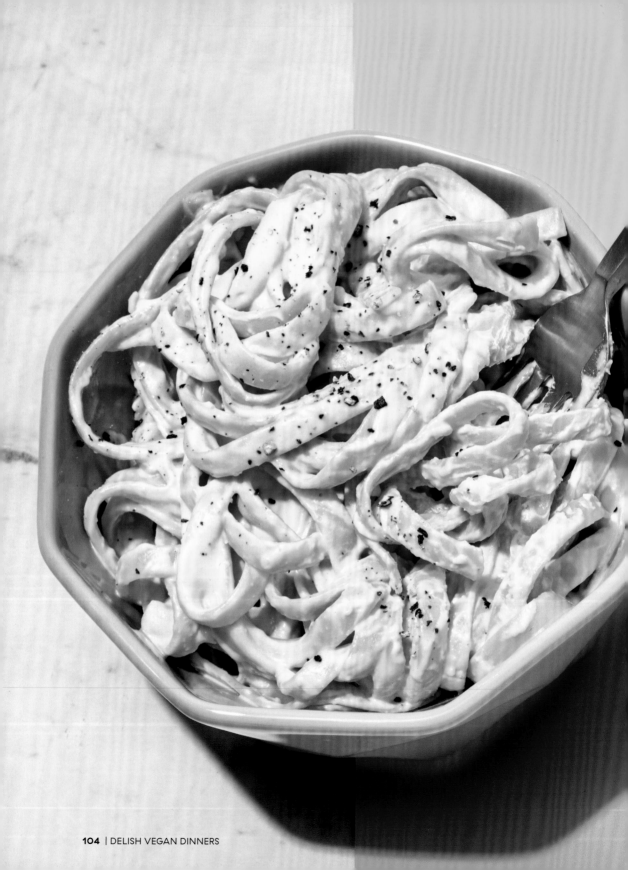

Cashew Cream Alfredo

 SERVES 3–4 | **TOTAL TIME: 4 HR 20 MIN**

Thanks to cashews, you can make an ultra-creamy, velvety smooth alfredo sauce *sans* dairy! Freshly cracked black pepper adds a burst of heat; if you're looking to add more fresh flavor, torn basil or parsley should do the trick.

1 cup raw unsalted cashews
1 pound fettuccine
2 garlic cloves, peeled
½ cup water, plus more as needed
¼ cup extra-virgin olive oil
¼ cup freshly grated vegan Parmesan
2 teaspoons nutritional yeast
Kosher salt
Freshly ground black pepper

1. In a medium bowl, add cashews and enough water to cover. Soak for 4 hours, or up to 12 hours, until they have softened. This will help to blend cashews into a fine paste. (If you don't have a high-powered blender, the closer to 12 hours the better.)

2. In a large pot of boiling salted water, cook pasta according to package instructions. Drain and set aside.

3. Blend cashews, garlic, ½ cup water, and olive oil on high for 1 to 2 minutes, or until mixture is completely smooth. Transfer mixture to a small saucepan and heat on medium-low for 1 minute, or until mixture is warm.

4. Add Parmesan and yeast, stirring to incorporate. If sauce is too thick, gradually add water, stirring to combine, until desired thickness is reached.

5. Season sauce to taste with salt and a generous amount of fresh black pepper. Add boiled pasta to sauce and toss to coat.

Meet Your New Favorite Curry

This hearty **Sesame Tofu Katsu Curry** brings ALL the textures, from crispy breading to silky sauce. A scoop of white rice is mandatory for soaking up every last drop.

TURN FOR THE RECIPE! →

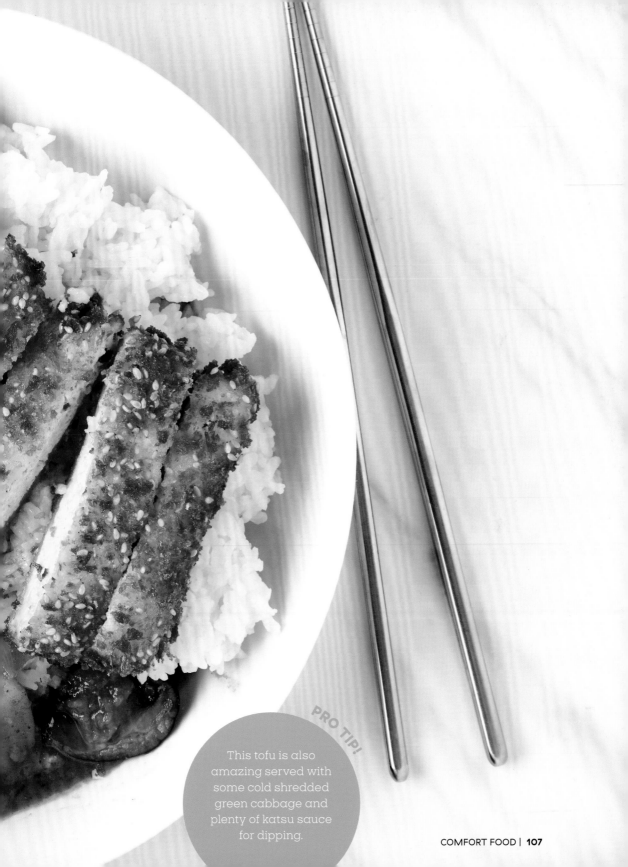

PRO TIP!

This tofu is also amazing served with some cold shredded green cabbage and plenty of katsu sauce for dipping.

Sesame Tofu Katsu Curry

SERVES 3–4 | **TOTAL TIME: 1 HR 20 MIN**

FOR THE CURRY ROUX

2 tablespoons extra-virgin olive oil
2 tablespoons all-purpose flour
2 tablespoons curry powder
1 teaspoon garam masala
1 teaspoon coriander powder
¼ teaspoon cayenne (optional)

FOR THE CURRY

2 tablespoons extra-virgin olive oil, divided
8 ounces baby bella mushrooms, halved
Kosher salt
1 small yellow onion, cut into large wedges
1 inch fresh ginger, peeled and thinly sliced
2 cups low-sodium vegetable broth or water
1 russet potato, peeled and cut into sixths
1 large carrot, cut into irregular chunks
1 medium Fuji apple, peeled and grated
2 small Roma tomatoes, chopped into large pieces
Low-sodium soy sauce

1. Make the curry roux: in a small saucepan over medium heat, heat 2 tablespoons olive oil. Add flour gradually, whisking to combine. Continue whisking constantly, until lightly golden and fragrant, 1 to 2 minutes. Stir in spices and cook for 30 seconds to 1 minute, until very fragrant, and then transfer mixture to a small bowl. (Mixture will be the texture of wet sand and will be very hot!)

2. Make the curry: in a large skillet over medium heat, heat 1 tablespoon olive oil. Add mushrooms in a single layer, cut side down. Cook undisturbed until cut sides are golden, about 4 minutes. Stir, season with salt, and cook 3 to 4 minutes more. Remove from heat.

3. Heat remaining tablespoon olive oil in a large pot over medium heat. Add onion, season with salt, and cook, stirring occasionally, until onion has softened slightly, 4 minutes. Add ginger and cook until fragrant, 1 minute.

4. Add broth and a big pinch of salt to pot with onions and bring to a boil, scraping bottom of pan with a wooden spoon to release any brown spots. Lower heat to a simmer and use a ladle to remove some hot broth or water. Transfer about one-quarter of curry roux to ladle and use chopsticks to stir until roux is dissolved into liquid. Add mixture back to pot and stir, then repeat process 3 more times until all roux is dissolved into pot. Add potato and simmer 5 minutes, partially covered.

5. Add carrots and half of grated apple and simmer partially covered, stirring occasionally, 8 to 10 minutes, or until carrots and potatoes are just tender. (If your vegetables aren't completely submerged in liquid, add more water or broth to cover.)

6. Stir in cooked mushrooms, tomatoes, and remaining

FOR THE TOFU KATSU

1 (14-ounce) block firm tofu,
   frozen in package for 24 hours
   and defrosted
Kosher salt
⅔ cup all-purpose flour
⅔ cup nondairy milk
¾ cup panko bread crumbs
1 tablespoon Dijon mustard
3 tablespoons sesame seeds
Vegetable oil, for frying
Cooked rice, for serving

apple, then season to taste with soy sauce.

7. Prepare the tofu: on a cutting board, sandwich tofu between doubled layers of paper towels and press down slowly with a flat-bottomed pan or second cutting board to remove moisture without cracking block.

8. Discard paper towel and stand up tofu on its short, small side. Slice tofu into 3 rectangular planks. Season each slice on all sides with salt.

9. Make breading station: Add flour to one shallow bowl, nondairy milk to another shallow bowl, and panko to a third. Whisk mustard into bowl with milk and sesame seeds into bowl with panko. Line a baking sheet with paper towels and fit with a metal cooling rack.

10. Bread tofu: Using one hand for dry breading and one hand for wet breading, coat one piece tofu in flour, then in milk mixture, then back in flour, back to milk, and finally into panko mixture, being sure to coat completely. Transfer breaded tofu to prepared rack and repeat with remaining tofu.

11. Heat about ½ inch vegetable oil in a large skillet over medium-high heat. When a piece of panko bubbles immediately when added to oil, add tofu. Cook until deeply golden on underside, 4 to 6 minutes. Flip and cook until golden on other side, 4 to 6 minutes more. Transfer to cooling rack and season with salt immediately.

12. To serve: Add rice and curry to each serving plate. Cut each piece of tofu into inch-wide strips and serve on top of curry and rice.

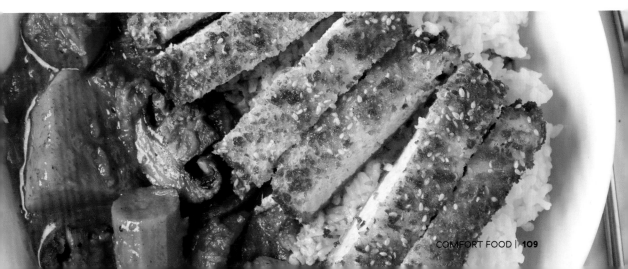

Chicken-Fried Mushrooms & Gravy

 SERVES 4 | 🕒 **TOTAL TIME: 30 MIN** |

Meaty oyster mushrooms stand in for steak in our indulgent take on this Southern classic. Buttermilk is a *must* for fried chicken, so we made our own with almond milk and vinegar.

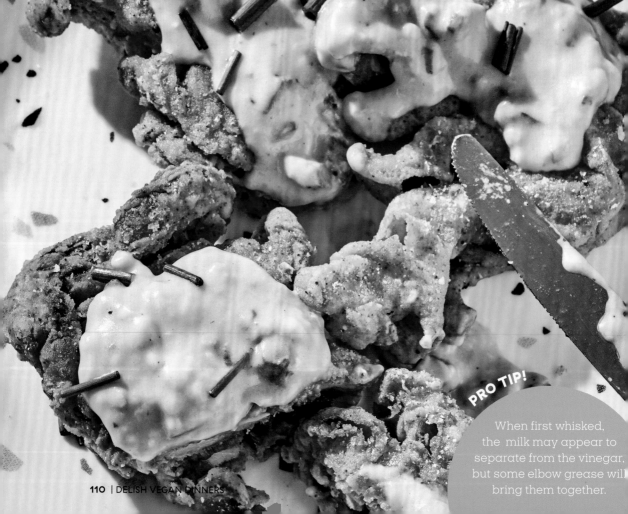

PRO TIP!

When first whisked, the milk may appear to separate from the vinegar, but some elbow grease will bring them together.

FOR THE CHICKEN–FRIED MUSHROOMS

2 large bunches oyster
   mushrooms (about 12 ounces)
2 cups all-purpose flour
2 tablespoons cornstarch
2 teaspoons sweet paprika
1 teaspoon garlic powder
1 teaspoon onion powder
½ teaspoon turmeric
Kosher salt
Freshly ground black pepper
1 cup unsweetened almond milk
1 tablespoon apple cider vinegar
Vegetable oil, for frying
Flaky sea salt

FOR THE GRAVY

2 tablespoons vegan butter
3 large cremini mushrooms (about
   3 ounces), chopped into small
   pieces
1 garlic clove, minced
2 tablespoons all-purpose flour
Vegetable oil, for frying
2 cups unsweetened almond milk
Chopped chives, for garnish

1. Make the chicken-fried mushrooms: Trim tough woody ends from oyster mushrooms, making sure to keep root intact. Slice bunches into thin planks, about ½-inch thick, lengthwise through root. Keep any pieces of mushroom that fall off of planks to batter separately.

2. In a shallow bowl, whisk together flour, cornstarch, paprika, garlic powder, onion powder, turmeric, ¾ teaspoon salt, and ¼ teaspoon pepper. In another shallow bowl, whisk almond milk with vinegar.

3. Toss one mushroom steak into flour mixture, making sure to coat spaces between mushrooms. Dip in almond milk. Repeat tossing in flour, dipping in almond milk, and tossing again in flour. Place on a plate. Repeat with remaining steaks and any extra mushroom bits.

4. Pour oil into a large cast-iron skillet until it is ½ inch deep. Heat over medium-high heat. When oil is hot and just starts to shimmer, reduce heat to medium and fry in 2 batches, turning once, until deep golden on both sides, about 8 minutes per side for large planks and 4 minutes per side for smaller pieces. Transfer to a paper-towel-lined plate and season with sea salt.

5. Meanwhile, make gravy: In a small saucepan, melt butter over medium-high heat. Add cremini mushrooms and cook, stirring occasionally, until mushrooms are golden, about 3 minutes. Add garlic and cook, stirring 1 minute, until fragrant.

6. Add flour to mushroom mixture and cook, stirring, 1 minute. While whisking, slowly pour almond milk into mushroom mixture. Bring to a boil, then reduce heat to medium and simmer, stirring, until gravy thickens, about 10 minutes. Season to taste with salt and pepper.

7. Arrange mushrooms on plates and pour gravy over top. Garnish with chives and more pepper.

Spiced Khichdi

 SERVES 4 | **TOTAL TIME: 1 HR 35 MIN**

The most basic version of this South Asian dish—composed only of rice, a pulse (like mung beans or lentils), turmeric, and salt—is an easy-to-digest Ayurvedic meal meant to balance all three doshas in the body. Depending on region, family, and cook, variations are endlessly diverse. Our version is loaded with warming spices and topped with addictive crispy fried garlic.

½ cup moong dal (split mung beans)

½ cup white rice

1 teaspoon fenugreek seeds

2 tablespoons coconut oil

6 cloves garlic, thinly sliced

½ teaspoon ajwain seeds

½ teaspoon nigella seeds

½ teaspoon cumin seeds

½ teaspoon fennel seeds

½ teaspoon ground coriander

½ teaspoon freshly ground black pepper

½ teaspoon ground cinnamon

¼ teaspoon ground white pepper

1 teaspoon ground turmeric

Pinch of asafetida (optional)

½-inch piece ginger, minced

1 teaspoon kala namak or kosher salt

1 small plum tomato, finely diced

4½ cups water, divided

Cilantro, for serving

1. In a large bowl, rinse moong dal and rice until water runs mostly clear, about 3 times. Add fenugreek and cover mixture with cold water by 2 inches. Let sit for 30 minutes to 1 hour.

2. In a medium pot over medium heat, heat oil. Add garlic and fry until lightly golden, stirring frequently to prevent burning, 2 to 3 minutes. Transfer garlic pieces to a plate and retain oil in pot.

3. Add all seeds, coriander, black pepper, cinnamon, white pepper, turmeric, asafetida (if using), ginger, and kala namak, stirring until toasty, about 1 minute. Add tomato and cook until pieces begin to fall apart, 4 minutes.

4. Add drained rice, moong dal, fenugreek, and 4 cups water and bring to a boil. Reduce heat to low, cover with a lid, and let simmer, stirring occasionally, until rice and dal are soft and falling apart, 25 minutes. Optionally, stir in remaining ½ cup water to loosen khichdi to desired consistency.

5. Serve with garlic chips and cilantro, if desired.

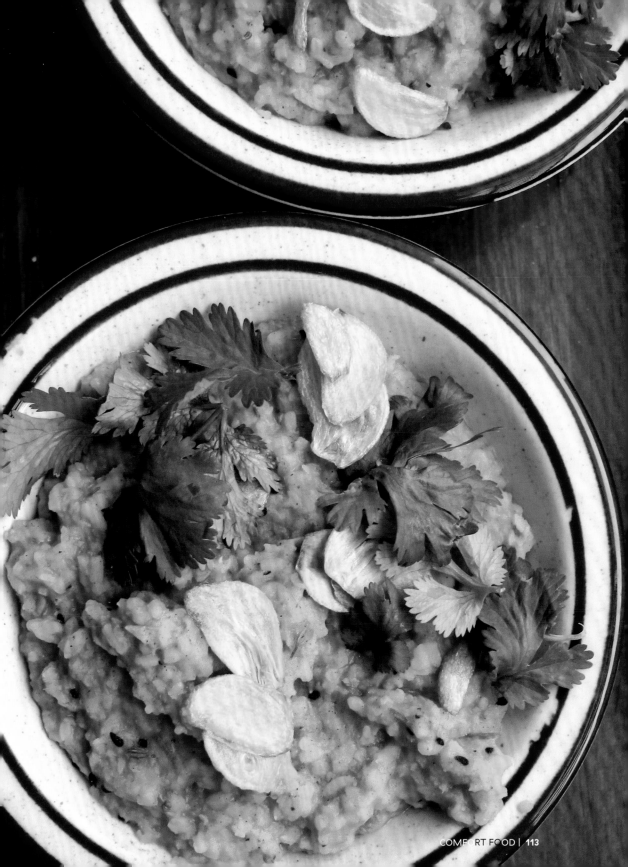

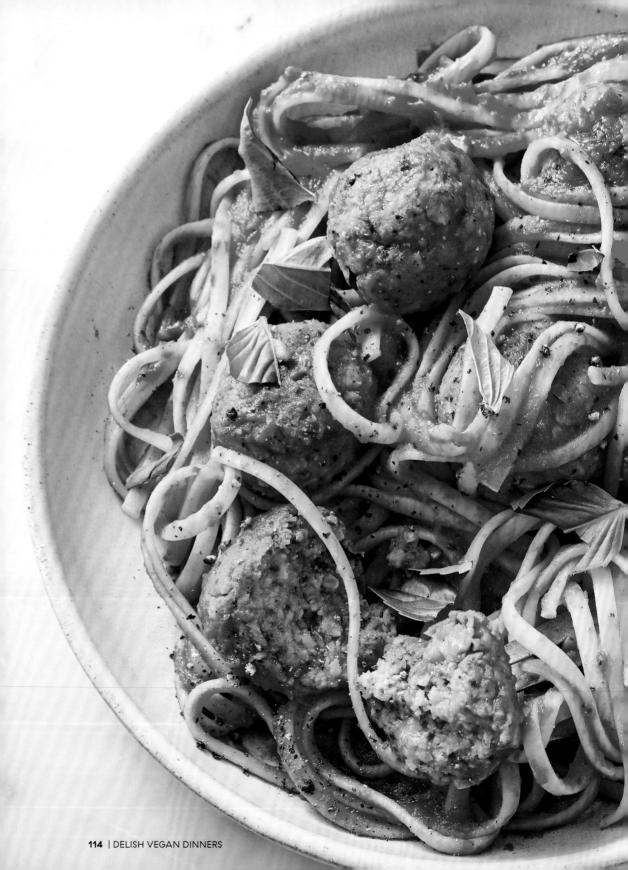

Best-Ever Chickpea "Meatballs"

 SERVES 3-4   **TOTAL TIME: 55 MIN**

These "meatballs" are reason 1,001 why we 🤍 chickpeas. Paired with smoky, savory fennel seeds, these little miracles taste surprisingly like their meat-based counterparts.

Cooking spray, for pan
2½ tablespoons chia seeds
6 tablespoons water
2 cups canned chickpeas
½ cup rolled oats
1½ tablespoons tomato paste
3 tablespoons chopped basil,
   plus more for serving
2 cloves garlic, minced
½ teaspoon fennel seeds
¼ teaspoon red pepper flakes
Kosher salt
Freshly ground black pepper
8 ounces dry pasta, such as
   spaghetti
12 ounces vegan marinara sauce

1. Preheat oven to 425°F and line a medium baking sheet with aluminum foil and grease with cooking spray.

2. In a medium bowl, stir together chia seeds and water. Let sit 5 minutes, until mixture gels and becomes thick.

3. Drain chickpeas, reserving liquid. Transfer chickpeas to a food processor and process until broken down but not smooth.

4. Add chia mixture, oats, tomato paste, basil, garlic, fennel seeds, and red pepper flakes to food processor and blend until combined. If mixture is too dry to hold together, add liquid from chickpea can 1 tablespoon at a time. Season with salt and pepper.

5. Form mixture into 16 balls and place on prepared baking sheet. Bake for 10 minutes, flip, and bake 8 to 10 minutes more, until golden and crisp.

6. In a large pot of boiling salted water, cook pasta according to package instructions and drain.

7. In a large skillet over medium heat, heat marinara sauce until warm. Add pasta and toss to combine with sauce. Serve pasta topped with meatballs and garnished with more basil.

Cincinnati-Style Chili Dogs

 SERVES 4–8 | TOTAL TIME: 1 HR 45 MIN

This rich, complex chili is so good, you'll want to put it on *way* more than just veggie dogs. We see chili mac, tamale pie, and plenty of chili fries in your future.

1 small onion, roughly chopped

1 stalk celery, roughly chopped

2 cloves garlic, peeled

2 tablespoons extra-virgin olive oil

½ tablespoon chili powder

1 teaspoon ground cumin

1 teaspoon ground cayenne

½ teaspoon smoked paprika

½ teaspoon ground coriander

½ teaspoon ground cinnamon

¼ teaspoon ground allspice

10 ounces cremini mushrooms, minced

1 tablespoon tomato paste

3 squares (20 grams) unsweetened baking chocolate

1 (14-ounce) can crushed tomatoes

2 cups low-sodium vegetable broth

½ tablespoon vegan Worcestershire sauce

Kosher salt

Freshly ground black pepper

8 vegan hot dogs

8 vegan hot dog buns, toasted

1 small white onion, chopped

Vegan cheddar, shredded (optional)

1. Make chili: Add onion, celery, and garlic to a food processor and puree until a paste forms. Heat olive oil in a medium heavy-bottomed pot over medium-high heat. Add vegetable puree and cook for 7 minutes, until mixture is fragrant. Add spices and stir until completely incorporated and cook for 30 seconds to toast the spices.

2. Reduce heat to medium and add mushrooms. Cook for 10 minutes, or until moisture has totally evaporated and mushrooms brown and begin to caramelize. Add tomato paste and chocolate, stirring until chocolate has melted and mushrooms are completely coated.

3. Pour in tomatoes, broth, and Worcestershire sauce and bring to a boil. Reduce heat to a simmer and cook uncovered for 1 hour for a looser, Cincinnati-style chili or 1½ hours for a thicker chili. Season to taste with salt and pepper.

4. Make chili hot dog: Over a medium-high grill or on a grill pan, grill hot dogs until they are heated through and charred. Move to toasted buns and cover with a layer of chili and a sprinkling of raw onion and vegan cheddar (if using).

PRO TIP!

Pile on the toppings! Try these with chopped jalapeño, sliced green onions, crushed chips, or diced avocado.

Chipotle "Queso" Crunchy Wraps

 SERVES 8 | **TOTAL TIME: 1 HR 15 MIN**

Recreate the joy of late night drive-through fast food in the comfort of your own kitchen! Opt for burrito-sized flour tortillas for easy folding.

Chipotle "Queso" (p. 10)
Lentil Filling (p. 80)
8 large flour tortillas
8 tostada shells
Guacamole
Shredded lettuce
Quartered cherry tomatoes
Vegetable oil, for pan

1. Build crunchwraps: Add a scoop of spiced lentils to the center of each flour tortilla, leaving a generous border clear for folding. Drizzle with chipotle "queso," then top with tostada shell. Spread tostada shell with an even layer of guacamole, then scatter lettuce and tomato on top.

2. Tightly fold edges of large tortilla toward the center, creating pleats. Carefully invert crunchwraps so pleats are on the bottom and they stay together.

3. In a skillet over medium heat, add crunchwrap seam-side down and cook until tortilla is golden, 3 minutes per side. Repeat with remaining crunchwraps.

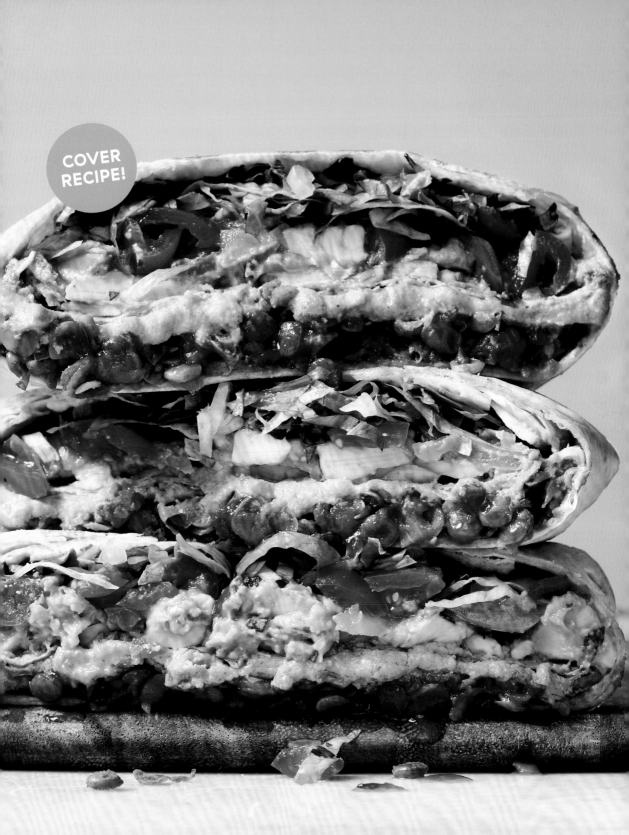

COVER RECIPE!

BBQ Tempeh Sandwiches

 SERVES 4 | **TOTAL TIME: 1 HR 10 MIN**

This smoky tempeh sandwich recipe is a cookout MVP. A homemade barbecue sauce made with bourbon and brown sugar is good enough to quit the store-bought stuff for good. Just add slaw and a toasty buttered bun!

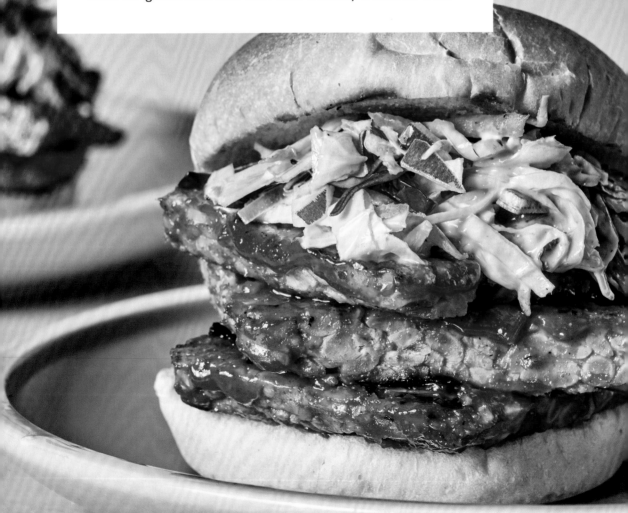

FOR THE BBQ TEMPEH

1 cup ketchup

¼ cup bourbon

3 tablespoons apple cider vinegar

⅓ cup packed brown sugar

¾ teaspoon smoked paprika

½ teaspoon onion powder

½ teaspoon garlic powder

¼ teaspoon ground mustard

2 (8-ounce) packages tempeh,
   cut crosswise into thirds, each
   third sliced lengthwise

Canola oil, for grilling

3 tablespoons vegan butter

4 vegan hamburger buns, split

FOR THE SLAW

½ cup vegan mayonnaise

4 teaspoons apple cider vinegar

½ teaspoon granulated sugar

¼ teaspoon celery seed

Kosher salt

Freshly ground black pepper

2 cups shredded green cabbage

1 cup shredded red cabbage

1 small carrot, coarsely grated

¼ small red onion, finely chopped

1. Make barbecue tempeh: Combine ketchup, bourbon, apple cider vinegar, brown sugar, paprika, onion powder, garlic powder, and ground mustard in a small saucepan. Place over medium heat and bring to a boil. Reduce heat to medium-low and simmer until sauce thickens and darkens in color, about 15 minutes. Pour BBQ sauce into a shallow baking dish.

2. Meanwhile, fill bottom of a medium saucepan with about 2 inches of water. Place saucepan over medium-high heat and bring to a simmer. Once simmering, arrange tempeh pieces evenly in a steamer basket. Set steamer basket in saucepan and cover. Reduce heat to medium and steam tempeh for 10 minutes.

3. Using tongs or a spatula, transfer tempeh from steamer basket directly into barbecue sauce. Toss to coat. Let marinate at least 30 minutes and up to overnight covered in refrigerator.

4. Preheat grill or grill pan to medium heat and oil grates. Spread butter on cut sides of buns. Remove tempeh from sauce, reserving any extra sauce. Arrange tempeh on grill and cook, turning occasionally, until lightly charred and warmed throughout, about 4 minutes per side.

5. Meanwhile, toast buns, cut-side down, on grill, about 3 minutes. Remove to a plate.

6. Meanwhile, make slaw: In a medium bowl, whisk vegan mayo with apple cider vinegar, granulated sugar, and celery seed. Season with salt and pepper. Add both cabbages, carrot, and red onion. Toss to coat.

7. Pile 3 pieces of tempeh on bottom buns and spoon reserved barbecue sauce over top. Pile slaw on top and close sandwich. Serve with any remaining slaw on side.

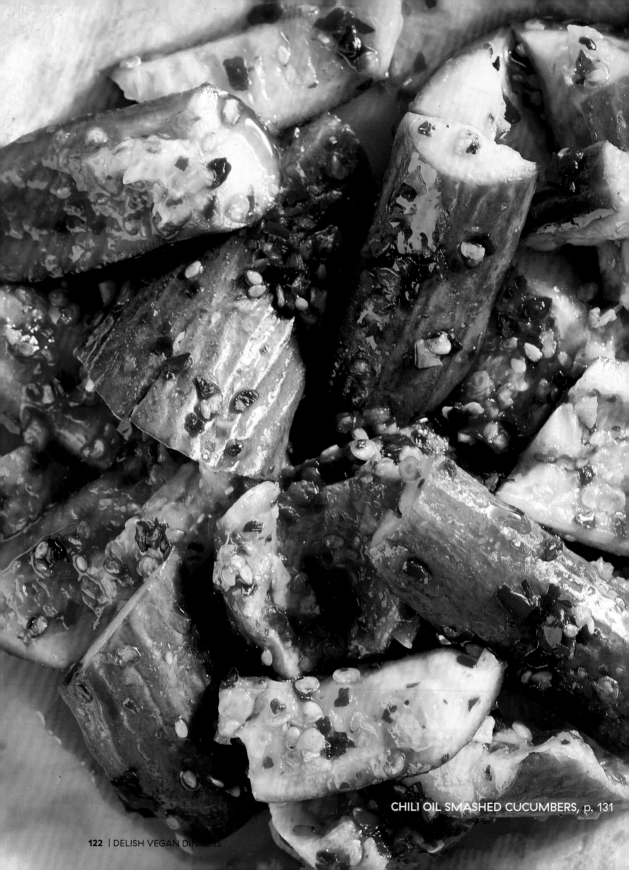

CHILI OIL SMASHED CUCUMBERS, p. 131

CHAPTER SIX

EXTRA VEGGIES

Sides and snacks that are ALL about the veg.

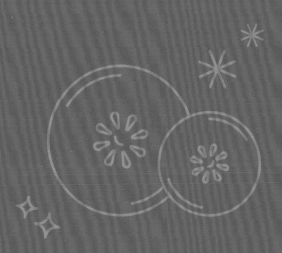

Mushroom "Calamari" with Spicy Marinara

SERVES 2-4 | **TOTAL TIME: 55 MIN**

Oyster mushrooms are lightly battered and fried in this squid-free take on the classic app. You can use other mushroom varieties, but the delicate "petals" of the oyster mushrooms are addictively crispy.

FOR THE SPICY MARINARA

2 tablespoons extra-virgin olive oil
2 cloves garlic, crushed
½ teaspoon red pepper flakes
1 tablespoon tomato paste
1 (14-ounce) can crushed
    tomatoes
¼ teaspoon dried oregano
2 tablespoons chopped fresh basil
    leaves (optional)
Kosher salt
Freshly ground black pepper

FOR THE "CALAMARI"

12 ounces oyster mushrooms
1 cup all-purpose flour
½ cup panko
1 teaspoon kosher salt
½ teaspoon freshly ground black
    pepper
1 teaspoon garlic powder
1 teaspoon smoked paprika
1 cup nondairy milk
¼ cup nondairy plain yogurt
Canola oil
Lemon wedges, for serving

1. Make spicy marinara: In a medium saucepan, heat olive oil over medium-low heat. Add garlic and red pepper flakes and cook, stirring, until garlic is soft, 3 to 4 minutes. Add tomato paste and cook, stirring, 1 minute. Add crushed tomatoes, oregano, and basil (if using). Bring to a simmer and cook 5 minutes; season to taste with salt and pepper. For a chunkier sauce, leave as is. For a smoother sauce, let cool slightly and transfer to a blender to puree.

2. Prepare calamari: Using your hands, pull apart mushrooms so they are separated into "petals." In a medium bowl, combine flour, panko, salt, pepper, garlic powder, and paprika. In another medium bowl, whisk nondairy milk and yogurt to combine.

3. Fit a deep skillet or pot with a thermometer and pour canola oil to come 3 inches up side of pot. Heat until thermometer registers 375°F.

4. Meanwhile, working in batches, dunk mushroom pieces in milk mixture, shaking off excess. Dredge in flour mixture, making sure pieces are evenly coated. Transfer to a lined baking sheet or plate and repeat until all pieces are coated.

5. Fry mushrooms in batches, 3 to 4 minutes, or until golden brown. Transfer to a paper towel to drain. While hot, sprinkle with salt. Serve with marinara and lemon wedges.

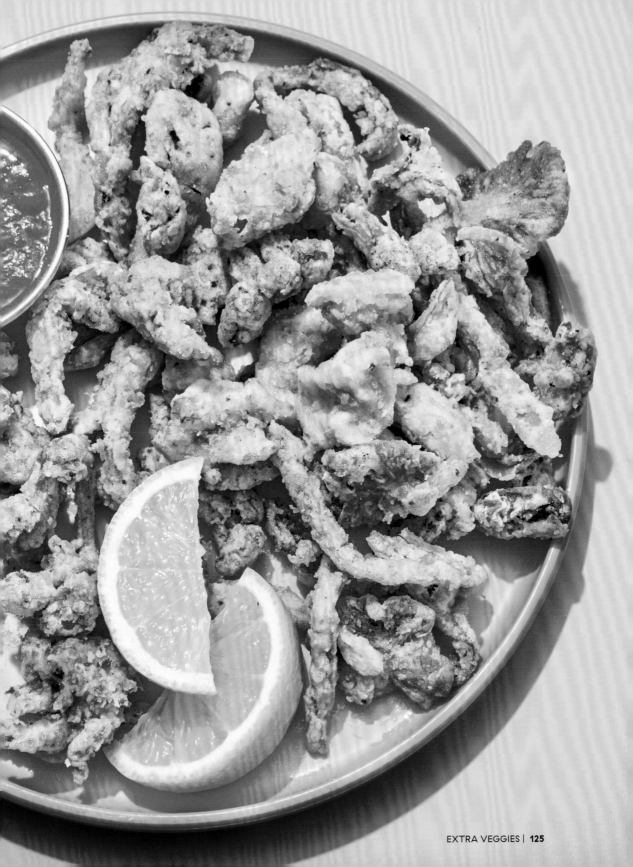

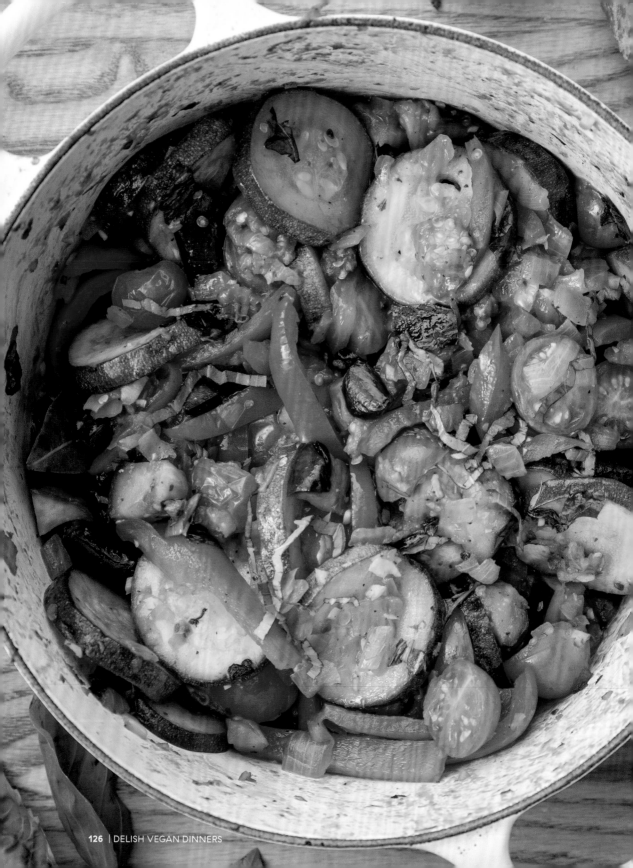

Ratatouille

You don't have to be a naturally talented rat–chef to make this inherently vegan French Provençal dish. The best ratatouille is made in the summer, when the veggies are at their peak, but thanks to always–decent cherry tomatoes, it can certainly be made year–round.

2 medium eggplants, diced into ½-inch pieces

Kosher salt

2 tablespoons extra-virgin olive oil, divided

Freshly ground black pepper

1 large onion, chopped

2 bell peppers, cut into ¼-inch spears

1 bay leaf

1 tablespoon tomato paste

½ cup dry white wine

2 zucchini, sliced into ¼-inch coins

3 cloves garlic

2 cups halved cherry tomatoes

1 teaspoon dried oregano

Pinch of crushed red pepper flakes

Bunch of fresh basil

Crusty baguette, for serving

1. Place eggplant in a colander and toss with a big pinch of salt. Let sit for about 20 minutes then pat eggplant dry to remove excess moisture.

2. In a Dutch oven (or a large pot), heat 1 tablespoon oil. Add eggplant and season with salt and pepper. Cook until golden, about 6 minutes, then remove eggplant.

3. Add remaining 1 tablespoon oil to pot. Add onion, bell peppers, and bay leaf and cook, stirring occasionally, until onion and peppers begin to turn tender, about 5 minutes.

4. Add tomato paste and stir until fragrant, about 1 minute, then deglaze pan with white wine and reduce until most of liquid has evaporated. Stir in zucchini and cook until tender, about 4 minutes. Stir in garlic, tomatoes, and oregano.

5. Season mixture with red pepper flakes, salt, and pepper and cook, stirring occasionally, until tomatoes start to break down.

6. Return eggplant to pot and stir to combine. Garnish with basil and serve warm or at room temperature with crusty baguette.

Kung Pao Brussels Sprouts

 SERVES 6 | **TOTAL TIME: 35 MIN**

Inspired by the popular Chinese takeout dish Kung Pao Chicken, these saucy Brussels are hard to stop eating. If you can't find whole chiles, add some heat with crushed red pepper flakes.

2 pounds Brussels sprouts, halved

2 tablespoons extra-virgin olive oil

Kosher salt

Freshly ground black pepper

1 tablespoon sesame oil

8 dried red chili peppers (optional)

2 cloves garlic, minced

1 tablespoon cornstarch

½ cup low-sodium soy sauce

½ cup water

2 teaspoons apple cider vinegar

1 tablespoon hoisin sauce

1 tablespoon packed brown sugar

2 teaspoons chili garlic sauce

Pinch of crushed red pepper flakes

Sesame seeds, for garnish

Green onions, thinly sliced, for garnish

Chopped roasted peanuts, for garnish

1. Preheat oven to 425°F. On a large, rimmed baking sheet, toss Brussels with olive oil and season with salt and pepper.

2. Bake until Brussels sprouts are tender and slightly crispy, about 20 minutes. Transfer Brussels sprouts to a large bowl (but keep baking sheet close). Preheat broiler.

3. In a small skillet over medium heat, heat sesame oil. Add chili peppers (if using) and garlic and cook, until fragrant, 1 minute. Stir in cornstarch. Add soy sauce, water, apple cider vinegar, hoisin sauce, brown sugar, and chili garlic sauce. Season with salt, pepper, and red pepper flakes. Bring mixture to a boil then reduce heat and simmer until thickened, about 3 minutes.

4. Pour sauce over Brussels sprouts and toss to combine. Return Brussels sprouts to baking sheet and broil until Brussels sprouts are glazed and sticky.

5. Garnish with sesame seeds, green onions, and peanuts before serving.

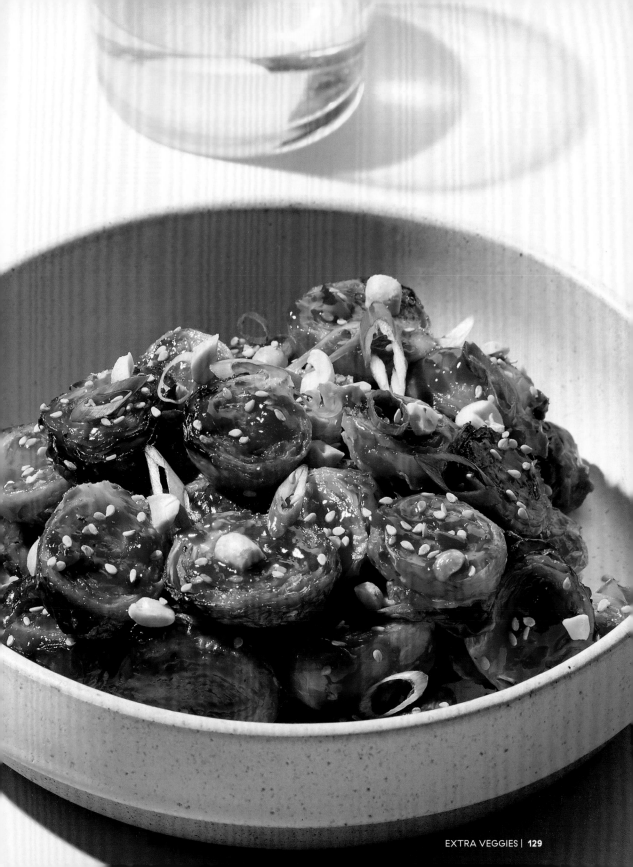

Chili Oil Smashed Cucumbers

 SERVES 2-4 | 🕐 **TOTAL TIME: 30 MIN**

The craggy, uneven texture of smashed cucumbers is just right for catching this crazy delicious homemade chili oil. You'll have plenty leftover to drizzle over soups, roasted veggies, avocado toast, or anything else that could use some kick.

FOR THE CHILI OIL

½ cup canola oil

1-inch piece ginger, minced

3 cloves garlic, minced

3 tablespoons ground chiles

2 teaspoons ground Szechuan peppercorns

1 tablespoon white sesame seeds

½ teaspoon MSG

¼ teaspoon kosher salt

FOR THE CUCUMBERS

6 Persian cucumbers

3 cloves garlic, grated

2 tablespoons prepared chili oil

1 tablespoon toasted sesame oil

½ teaspoon MSG

Kosher salt

1. Make chili oil: In a small pot, heat oil until starting to smoke then remove from heat.

2. Meanwhile, in a medium heatproof bowl or jar, whisk to combine all other ingredients. Slowly pour hot oil over spices, letting it sizzle through evenly, streaming gradually and carefully. Whisk to incorporate fully and let cool completely.

3. Prepare cucumbers: Cut each cucumber into thirds, then use knife to smash each piece into 2 craggy halves.

4. In a large bowl, toss smashed cucumbers with chili oil, sesame oil, and MSG until evenly combined. Season with salt to taste.

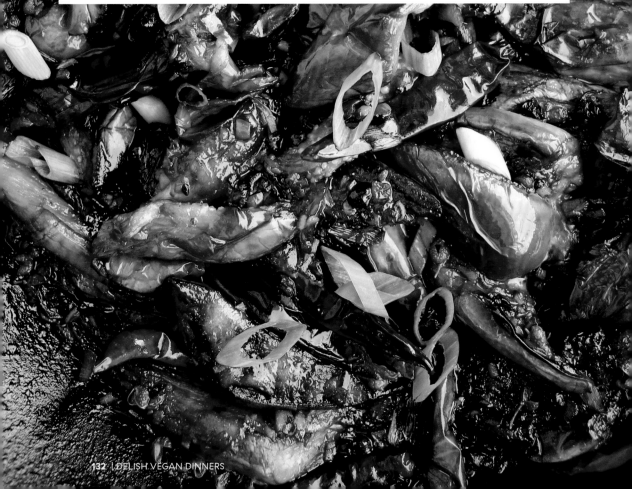

Sichuan-Style "Fish Fragrant" Eggplant

 SERVES 4 | **TOTAL TIME: 50 MIN**

Originating from the Sichuan province in China, 魚香 (yu xiang) literally means "fish fragrance" and describes a flavor profile originally used to prepare regional fish dishes. This punchy but harmoniously savory spice combination grew in popularity and is now used to season vegetable stir fries and meat stews.

- 3 Chinese eggplants (about 1¼ pounds), halved lengthwise and cut into thick diagonal strips
- 2 teaspoons kosher salt
- 3 tablespoons cornstarch
- Canola oil
- 1 teaspoon ground Sichuan peppercorn (optional)
- 6 to 12 dried red chiles (optional)
- 1 tablespoon chopped pickled chile, sambal oelek, or freshly sliced Thai chiles
- 3 tablespoons fermented chile bean paste
- 1 head garlic, minced, divided
- 1 tablespoon minced fresh ginger
- ½ teaspoon ground white pepper
- 3 green onions, thinly sliced, divided
- 1½ tablespoons low-sodium soy sauce
- 1½ tablespoons rice wine vinegar
- 2 teaspoons Chinese black vinegar
- 4 teaspoons granulated sugar
- ½ teaspoon MSG (optional)
- ½ cup water or low-sodium vegetable broth
- 2 teaspoons toasted sesame oil
- Cooked rice, for serving

1. In a large bowl, toss eggplant evenly with salt. Let sit for 20 to 30 minutes, then gently squeeze out as much moisture as possible. Drain and pat dry with a paper towel. Transfer to a dry bowl or sheet tray then add cornstarch and toss to coat eggplant evenly.

2. In a large skillet over medium heat, heat skillet for 1 minute then heat 2 tablespoons oil until it starts to smoke slightly. Working in batches to avoid overcrowding pan, fry eggplant until lightly golden on all sides, 3 to 4 minutes. Transfer to a bowl and set aside. Repeat with remaining eggplant, adding more oil as necessary if pan begins to run dry.

3. Return empty skillet to medium-low heat and add 2 tablespoons oil. Add Sichuan peppercorn, chiles, bean paste, half the garlic, ginger, white pepper, and half the green onions. Stirring constantly, cook until fragrant and garlic is barely golden, about 1 minute.

4. Return eggplant to skillet. Pour in soy sauce, vinegars, sugar, MSG (if using), and water or broth, stirring occasionally until mixture thickens and becomes glossy. Stir in sesame oil, remaining garlic, and remaining green onions in final minute of cooking.

5. Serve with rice, if desired.

PRO TIP!

We love using a small amount of MSG to add a boost of sweet and savory umami to dishes, including this eggplant.

Giardiniera

🍴 MAKES: 3 PINT JARS	TOTAL TIME: 1 HR 15 MIN	

This pickled Italian relish is endlessly versatile. Try it on sandwiches, tossed into a hearty salad, or in place of olives in your martini. Serrano peppers can be *very* spicy, so opt for a pinch of red pepper flakes instead if you're heat-averse.

½ small (about 2-pound) head cauliflower, cut into small florets

2 medium carrots, peeled and cut into ¼-inch coins

2 stalks celery, sliced into ¼-inch pieces

1 red bell pepper, chopped large

2 cloves garlic, sliced thin

1 serrano pepper, sliced thin

2 cups white wine vinegar

1 cup water

1½ tablespoons granulated sugar

1 tablespoon kosher salt

2 bay leaves

2 teaspoons fennel seeds

2 teaspoons coriander seeds

2 teaspoons dried oregano

1. Combine cauliflower, carrots, celery, bell pepper, garlic, and serrano pepper in a large bowl. Toss to combine then pack into glass jars.

2. In a medium saucepan over medium heat, combine vinegar, water, sugar, salt, bay leaves, fennel seeds, coriander seeds, and dried oregano. Stir to dissolve salt and sugar and bring to a boil.

3. When mixture is boiling, remove from heat, remove bay leaves, and pour mixture over jarred vegetables. Let cool completely, place lids on jars, and refrigerate. Giardinara will last at least 1 week in fridge.

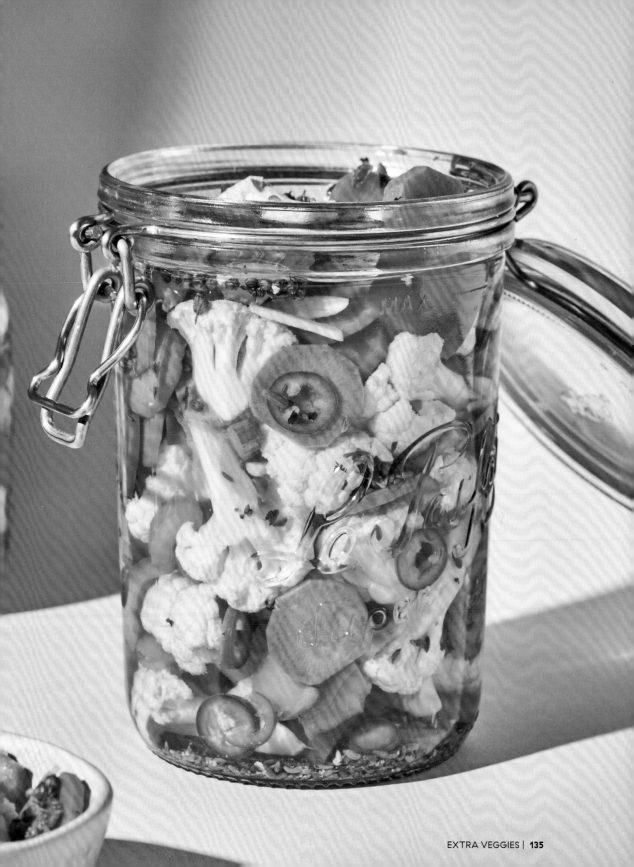

BBQ Braised Kale

 SERVES 4–6 | TOTAL TIME: 1 HR 5 MIN

Inspired by the delicious smoky greens that often come with a good barbecue brisket platter, this kale is like nothing you've had before.

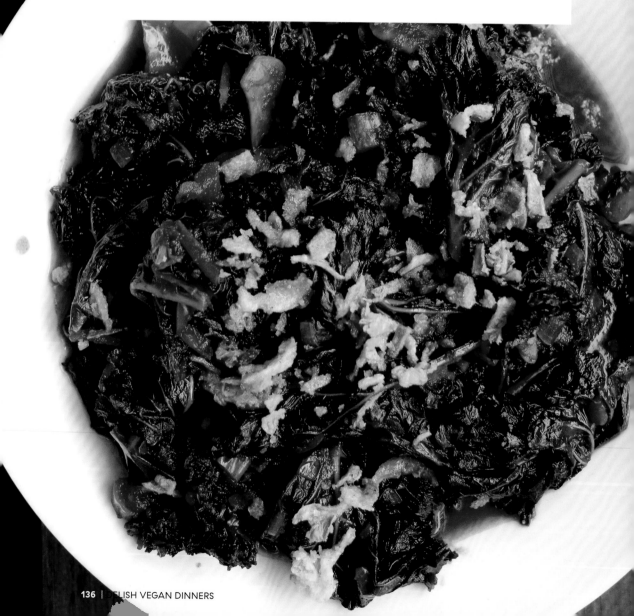

FOR THE BARBECUE SAUCE

⅔ cup tomato paste

3 tablespoons granulated sugar

¼ cup apple cider vinegar

Juice of 1 lime

½ teaspoon kosher salt

1 tablespoon dark soy sauce

¼ cup packed brown sugar

2 tablespoons balsamic vinegar

½ teaspoon smoked paprika

½ teaspoon onion powder

½ teaspoon garlic powder

½ teaspoon ground mustard

1 teaspoon freshly ground black
  pepper

Pinch of ground cumin (optional)

2 cloves garlic, grated

FOR THE KALE

1 pound kale, thoroughly rinsed
  and patted dry (8 large leaves)

3 tablespoons coconut oil, divided

1 teaspoon gochugaru or ½
  teaspoon crushed red pepper
  flakes

4 cloves garlic, thinly sliced

1 small onion, finely diced

1 plum tomato, finely diced

1 Cubanelle pepper, thinly sliced
  into rings

½ teaspoon kosher salt

2 cups low-sodium vegetable
  broth or water

Fried onions, for topping

1. Make barbecue sauce: In a large bowl, stir together all ingredients until smooth.

2. Strip leafy kale from stalky stems. Tear leaves into 2-inch pieces and finely chop stems into ⅓-inch pieces. Keep separate.

3. In a large pot over medium heat, heat 2 tablespoons oil. Add gochugaru and garlic and stir until fragrant, 30 seconds. Increase heat to medium-high then add onion, tomato, pepper, kale stems, and salt. Cook and stir until tomatoes begin to caramelize, 10 to 12 minutes.

4. Add remaining 1 tablespoon oil, then add kale leaves in 2 batches, allowing first batch to wilt before adding second. Once kale is fully wilted, about 6 minutes, add broth and use a wooden spoon to scrape and deglaze the pan. Bring to a simmer, then add 1 cup barbecue sauce, stirring to combine evenly.

5. Cover pot with lid, reduce heat to low, and gently simmer until kale is completely tender, about 25 minutes.

6. Top with fried onions before serving.

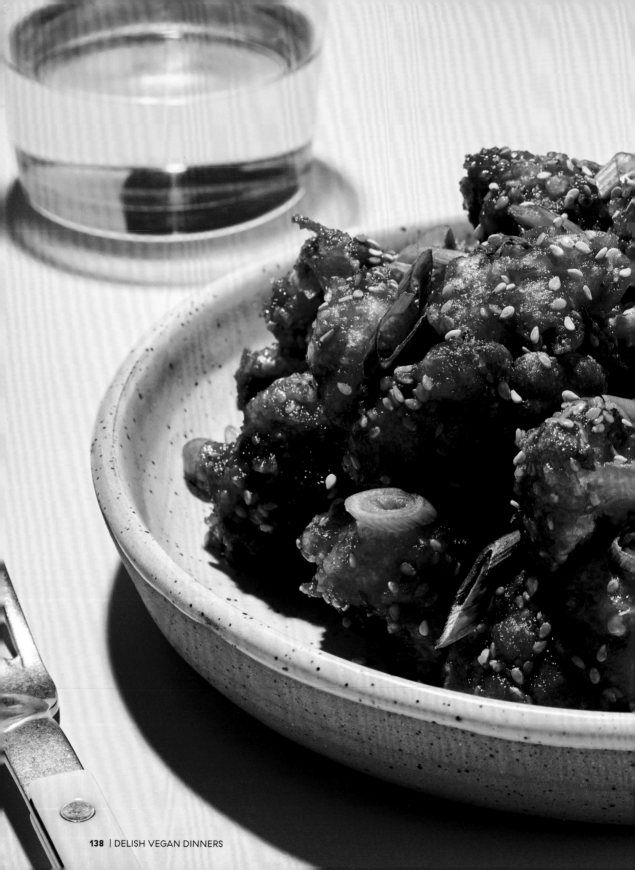

Chili Garlic Fried Cauliflower

 SERVES 6 **TOTAL TIME: 35 MIN**

Cauliflower florets are battered in a tempura–like batter, creating a light, crispy coating. Eat these babies ASAP, while they're still hot, for maximum crunch.

½ cup all-purpose flour, sifted

½ cup cornstarch

1 teaspoon baking powder

1 cup ice water

Kosher salt

Vegetable oil, for frying

1 head cauliflower, cut into florets

⅓ cup chili garlic sauce

2 tablespoons low-sodium soy sauce

3 tablespoons brown sugar

2 teaspoons sesame oil

1 teaspoon grated ginger

2 tablespoons sesame seeds

2 green onions, thinly sliced

1. In a large bowl, whisk together flour, cornstarch, and baking powder. Add ice water and 1 teaspoon salt, and stir to combine. The batter should be thin.

2. In a large skillet over medium heat, heat about ¼ inch vegetable oil until oil is shimmering. Toss cauliflower in batter until fully coated. Working in batches, add cauliflower and cook until golden on all sides, about 4 minutes per side. Drain on paper towels and season with more salt, if necessary.

3. In a medium bowl, whisk together chili garlic sauce, soy sauce, brown sugar, sesame oil, and ginger. Toss fried cauliflower in sauce. Sprinkle with sesame seeds and green onions and serve.

Miso Maple Glazed Carrots

 SERVES 4 | ⏱ **TOTAL TIME: 50 MIN**

These sweet–savory carrots are topped with the most delicious mix of crunchy nuts and spices. It's easy enough to chop the nuts by hand and smash the coriander seeds with the back of a knife, but you can also pulse everything in a food processor or grind them up with a mortar and pestle.

⅓ cup pure maple syrup

2 tablespoons white miso paste

2 tablespoons extra-virgin olive oil

2 tablespoons packed brown sugar

Large pinch of crushed red pepper flakes

2 pounds whole carrots, scrubbed and halved crosswise, halved lengthwise as well if large

Kosher salt

1 tablespoon fresh lemon juice

⅓ cup toasted pistachios, chopped

1 teaspoon black sesame seeds

1 teaspoon white sesame seeds

1 teaspoon coriander seeds, crushed

¼ teaspoon smoked paprika

Flaky sea salt

1. Preheat oven to 425°F. In a small bowl, whisk together maple syrup, white miso paste, oil, brown sugar, and red pepper flakes.

2. Line a large, rimmed baking sheet with foil. Arrange carrots on baking sheet and drizzle maple syrup mixture over top. Season with salt, toss to coat, and spread evenly on baking sheet.

3. Bake, tossing halfway through, until carrots are tender and glaze is thickened and caramelized in places, about 35 to 40 minutes.

4. Remove baking sheet from oven and carefully sprinkle carrots with lemon juice; toss to coat.

5. In another small bowl, combine pistachios, sesame seeds, coriander, and paprika.

6. Transfer roasted carrots to a platter, scraping any glaze remaining on sheet tray over top. Let cool slightly. Sprinkle with pistachio mixture, more red pepper flakes, if desired, and flaky sea salt. Serve warm or at room temperature.

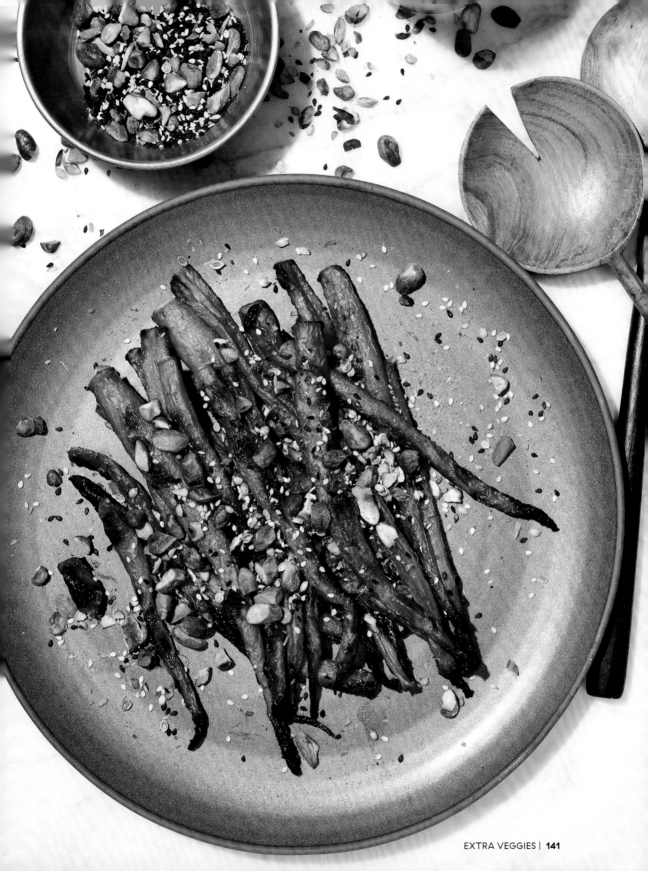

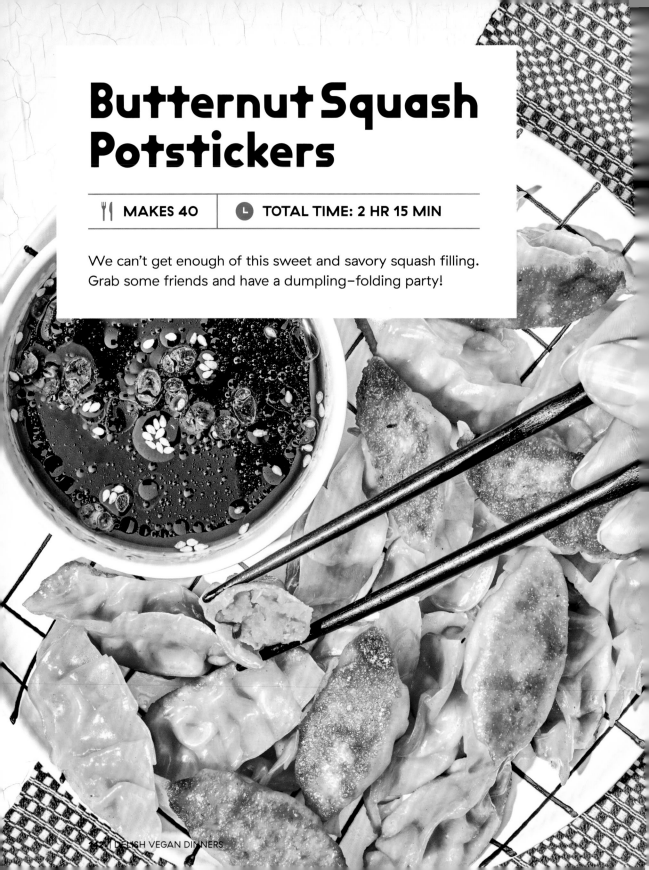

Butternut Squash Potstickers

🍴 **MAKES 40** | 🕐 **TOTAL TIME: 2 HR 15 MIN**

We can't get enough of this sweet and savory squash filling. Grab some friends and have a dumpling–folding party!

FOR THE POTSTICKERS

1 butternut squash (about
   2 pounds)
2 teaspoons extra-virgin olive oil
Kosher salt
Freshly ground black pepper
1 tablespoon minced ginger
3 cloves garlic, minced
3 green onions, thinly sliced
1 tablespoon low-sodium soy
   sauce
1 tablespoon rice wine vinegar
¼ teaspoon crushed red pepper
   flakes
40 dumpling wrappers
2 tablespoons vegetable oil,
   for cooking

FOR THE DIPPING SAUCE

¼ cup low-sodium soy sauce
1 tablespoon rice wine vinegar
1 teaspoon sesame oil
1 green onion, thinly sliced
1 teaspoon toasted sesame seeds

1. Preheat oven to 450°F and line a small baking sheet with parchment paper. Cut ends off squash then cut in half lengthwise and scoop out seeds. Drizzle olive oil over squash and season with salt and pepper. Place squash, cut-side down, on prepared baking sheet and bake until a knife inserted in the thickest part meets no resistance, about 40 minutes. Let cool.

2. When squash is cool enough to handle, scoop flesh into a large bowl and mash with a fork until smooth. You should have about 2 cups of puree.

3. Add ginger, garlic, green onions, soy sauce, vinegar, and red pepper flakes to squash and stir to combine. Taste and season with salt and pepper to taste.

4. Fill a small bowl with water. Work with one wrapper at a time and keep remaining wrappers covered with a damp paper towel. Place a wrapper on a clean surface and place a heaping teaspoon of filling in center. Dip your finger in water and wet all edges of wrapper.

5. Seal wrapper together by making folds starting on one end and working your way toward other end. Use more water to help seal dumplings tightly. Repeat with remaining wrappers and filling.

6. In a large skillet over medium-high heat, heat 2 tablespoons vegetable oil. Add potstickers, seam-side up, in a single layer, working in batches as needed. Sear for 2 minutes, or until bottoms are golden. Reduce heat to low and very carefully add ¼ cup water (it will splatter!). Cover with a lid and let steam for 5 minutes, or until wrappers are soft. Remove from pan, carefully wipe pan dry, and repeat with remaining potstickers.

7. Make dipping sauce: In a small bowl, combine all ingredients. Serve potstickers with dipping sauce.

Gamja Jorim

🍴 SERVES 4	🕐 TOTAL TIME: 40 MIN	

Gamja jorim—"gamja" meaning potatoes and "jorim" meaning braised or simmered—is a cozy Korean dish made of potatoes simmered in a broth seasoned with soy sauce, honey or rice syrup, and gochugaru if spiciness is desired. It's simple and inexpensive to make at home and even easier to enjoy. Eat it with rice as a low-maintenance weeknight dinner or serve it alongside your main course.

2 tablespoons grapeseed oil
1 pound baby potatoes, halved
Kosher salt
1 medium yellow onion, diced
4 cloves garlic, minced
1 cup water or low-sodium
   vegetable broth
¼ cup low-sodium soy sauce
1 tablespoon rice wine vinegar
3 tablespoons corn syrup
2 teaspoons gochugaru (optional)
1 carrot, finely diced
2 teaspoons toasted sesame oil
1 green onion, thinly sliced,
   plus more for garnish
Sesame seeds, for garnish

1. In a large skillet over medium heat, heat oil. Add potatoes, season with a large pinch of salt, and let cook until a golden crust develops, stirring occasionally, 8 to 10 minutes. Add onion and garlic and stir until garlic is golden, 2 to 3 minutes. Add water, soy sauce, vinegar, corn syrup, and gochugaru (if using), then stir to evenly combine. Bring to a simmer and let cook for 8 minutes.

2. Add carrots then continue cooking until liquid has reduced to a sticky sauce, stirring occasionally, about 4 minutes. Remove from heat, add sesame oil and green onions, and stir to combine evenly.

3. Garnish with more green onions and sesame seeds before serving.

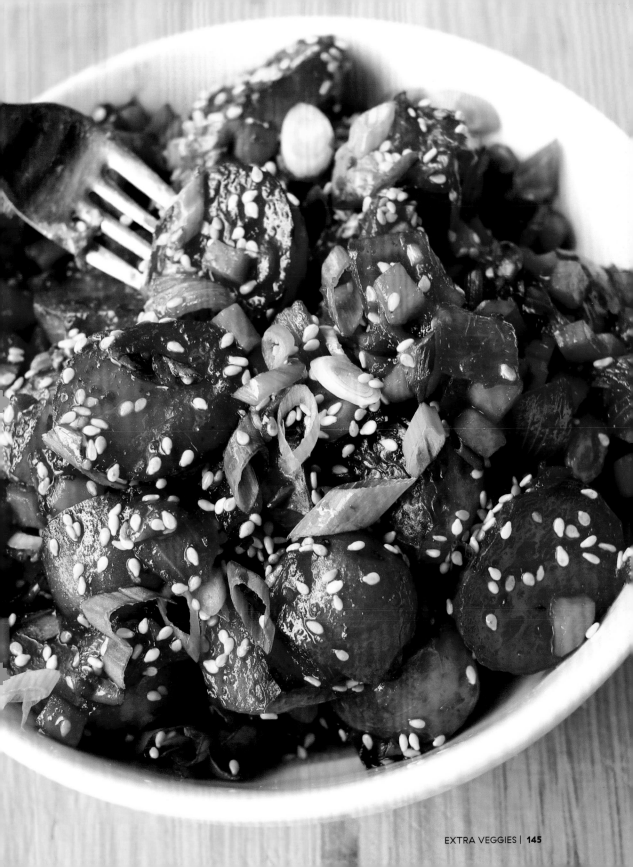

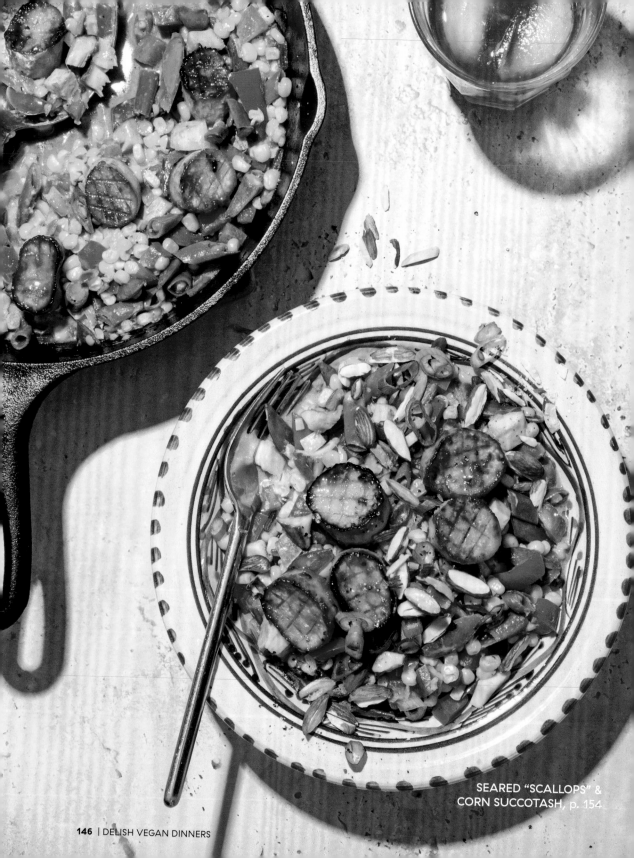

SEARED "SCALLOPS" &
CORN SUCCOTASH, p. 154

CHAPTER SEVEN

WEEKENDS & SPECIAL OCCASIONS

Extra-special eats for date nights, dinner parties, holidays, and everything in between.

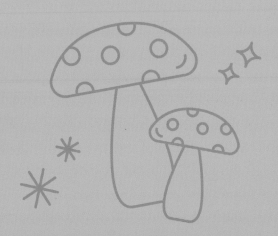

Polenta with Wild Mushroom Ragu

 SERVES 4–6   **TOTAL TIME: 1 HR 35 MIN**

Make this showstopper with a custom blend of your favorite funghi. If wild mushrooms aren't available, creminis or button mushrooms are perfect subs.

FOR THE RAGU

1 ounce dried porcini mushrooms
2 tablespoons extra-virgin olive oil
2 shallots, finely chopped
2 garlic cloves, very thinly sliced
2 pounds mixed wild mushrooms
 (such as shiitake, trumpet,
 oyster), trimmed and coarsely
 chopped
1 tablespoon chopped fresh
 tarragon, plus more for serving
2 bay leaves
1½ teaspoons kosher salt, plus
 more to taste
2 teaspoons all-purpose flour
½ cup red wine

FOR THE POLENTA

4 cups vegetable broth
4 cups water
2 cups polenta
3 tablespoons vegan butter
½ cup nutritional yeast

1. Place the dried porcinis in a medium bowl and cover with 2 cups of boiling water. Let soak 30 minutes. Strain liquid into a glass measuring cup, pressing on mushrooms to release liquid. Reserve liquid and coarsely chop mushrooms; set aside.

2. In a large skillet, heat oil over medium heat. Add shallots and cook, stirring, until softened, 3 to 4 minutes. Add garlic and cook until softened, 2 minutes. Add mushrooms, tarragon, bay leaves, and ½ teaspoon salt. Increase heat to medium-high and cook until mushrooms are tender and liquid is evaporated, 4 to 5 minutes.

3. Add flour and cook, stirring constantly, 2 minutes. Add porcini mushrooms and wine and increase heat to high. Cook until liquid has mostly evaporated into a glaze, scraping any bits on bottom of pan. Add porcini soaking liquid and bring to a simmer. Cook on medium-high 10 to 15 minutes, or until broth is thick and flavorful. Salt to taste and remove bay leaves before serving.

4. To make polenta: In a large heavy saucepan, bring broth and water to a boil. Add 1 teaspoon salt and gradually whisk in polenta. Reduce heat to low and cook, stirring often with a wooden spoon, until thickened to your liking, about 15 minutes. Stir in vegan butter and nutritional yeast until melted. Serve immediately with mushroom ragu. Garnish with chopped tarragon.

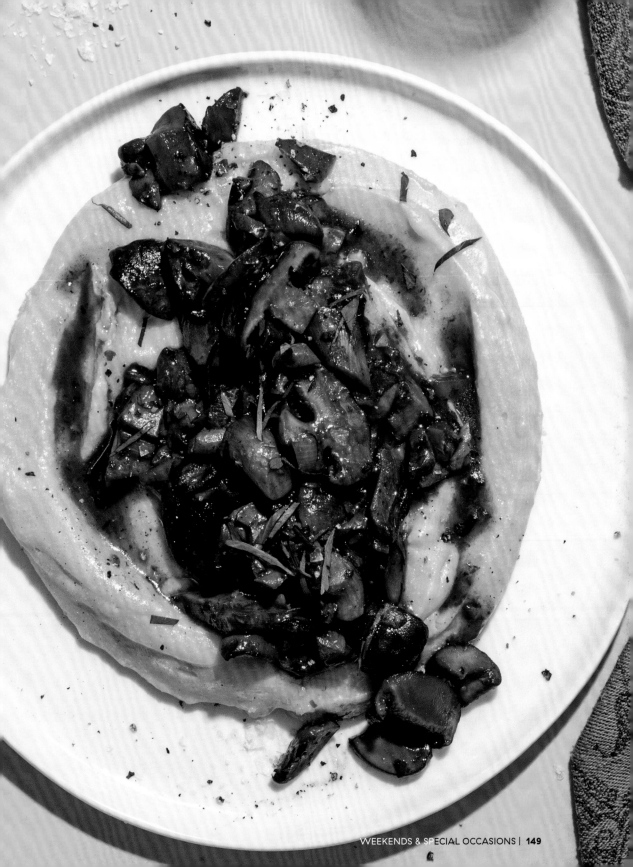

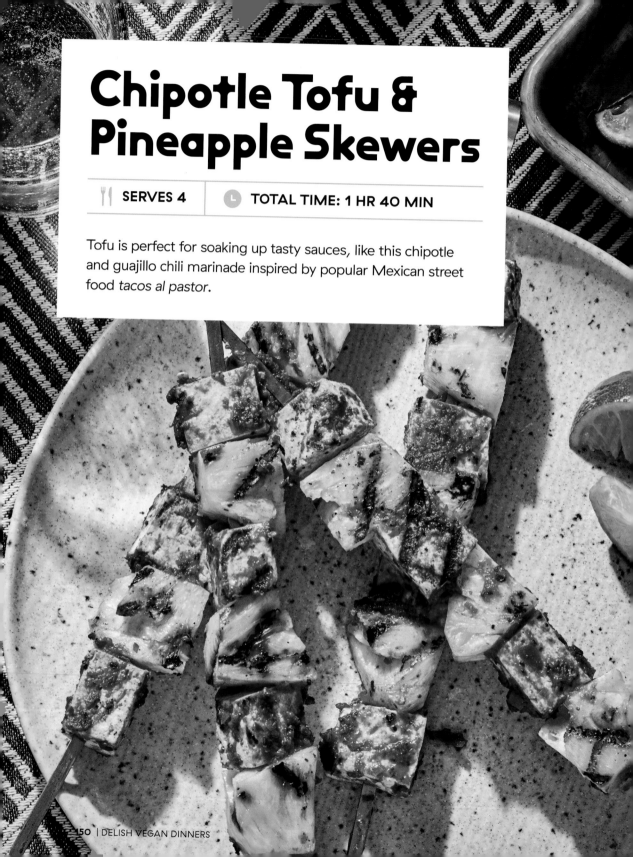

Chipotle Tofu & Pineapple Skewers

🍴 **SERVES 4** | 🕐 **TOTAL TIME: 1 HR 40 MIN**

Tofu is perfect for soaking up tasty sauces, like this chipotle and guajillo chili marinade inspired by popular Mexican street food *tacos al pastor*.

1 pound firm or extra-firm tofu, drained and cut into 1-inch cubes

3 guajillo chiles, stems and seeds removed and torn into small pieces

1 cup boiling water

½ medium white onion, half roughly chopped, half finely chopped, divided

¼ cup white vinegar

4 garlic cloves

1 tablespoon annatto paste (also called achiote paste)

1 chopped chipotle chile en adobo

2 teaspoons dried oregano

1½ teaspoons sugar

¼ cup extra-virgin olive oil

3 cups pineapple chunks (cut into 1-inch cubes)

Lime wedges, for serving

1. Arrange tofu cubes in a single layer on a rimmed baking sheet lined with several sheets of paper towel. Place more paper towels on top of tofu and another rimmed baking sheet. Weight top baking sheet with a few heavy books or cans. Let drain, changing paper towels when saturated with water, at least 30 minutes or up to overnight in refrigerator.

2. Meanwhile, in a medium heatproof bowl, cover guajillo chiles with boiling water and soak 15 minutes until chiles are softened. Drain.

3. Place drained chiles into a blender and add onion, vinegar, garlic, annatto paste, chipotle, oregano, and sugar. Pulse until pureed.

4. Heat a large skillet over medium and add olive oil. Pour in chile puree and cook, stirring constantly, until puree thickens and darkens slightly in color, about 5 minutes. Pour marinade into a heatproof medium shallow bowl or baking dish. Add drained tofu to bowl with marinade and toss to coat. Let marinate, turning tofu a few times, for at least 30 minutes and up to 2 hours refrigerated.

5. Alternate marinated tofu with pineapple chunks on 10-inch skewers. Reserve extra marinade for serving.

6. Preheat grill or grill pan to medium heat. Arrange skewers evenly on grill and cook, turning every few minutes, until tofu is golden and pineapple is lightly charred, about 10 minutes total. Remove from grill and serve with lime wedges and extra marinade as a salsa.

PRO TIP!

Wooden skewers tend to burn over a hot grill. If using, soak wooden skewers in water for 30 minutes before adding your tofu and pineapple.

Veggie Paella (Paella Verdura)

🍴 SERVES 4–5	🕐 TOTAL TIME: 50 MIN

This veggie-packed paella comes together in under an hour, and, even better, most of the cooking happens in the oven. Briefly returning the skillet to the stovetop after baking is the key to achieving a crispy rice crust on the bottom, often referred to as *socarrat* (meaning "burnt" in Catalan).

4 tablespoons extra-virgin olive oil, divided

2 medium zucchini, sliced into half moons

8 ounces sliced mushrooms

Kosher salt

½ small yellow onion, finely chopped

3 cloves garlic, finely chopped

1 teaspoon smoked paprika

1 pinch saffron threads (optional)

1 (14-ounce) can chopped tomatoes

1½ cups short grain paella rice (such as Bomba rice)

1 cup fresh or frozen peas

1 cup piquillo peppers, sliced (or roasted red peppers)

5 ounces baby spinach

3½ cups vegetable broth

Chopped parsley, for serving

Lemon wedges, for serving

1. Preheat oven to 425°F.

2. In a deep 12-inch cast-iron or ovenproof skillet, heat 2 tablespoons oil over medium heat. Add zucchini, mushrooms, and pinch of salt. Cook, undisturbed, until golden on one side, about 3 minutes. Continue cooking, stirring until golden and tender. Transfer to a small bowl.

3. To same pan, add 2 tablespoons olive oil and return to medium heat. Add onion and pinch of salt and cook, stirring, until softened, 3 to 5 minutes. Add garlic, smoked paprika, and saffron if using, and cook, stirring, until fragrant, 30 seconds. Add tomatoes and rice, stirring to coat. Stir in zucchini mixture, peas, piquillo peppers, and spinach, stirring to wilt spinach. Add broth and ¾ teaspoon salt, then bring to a boil. Transfer to oven and bake, uncovered and undisturbed, until rice is tender and liquid is absorbed, 20 to 22 minutes.

4. Transfer to stovetop and finish cooking on medium heat 2 to 3 minutes to crisp up rice; let rest 5 minutes. Garnish with chopped parsley and serve with lemon wedges.

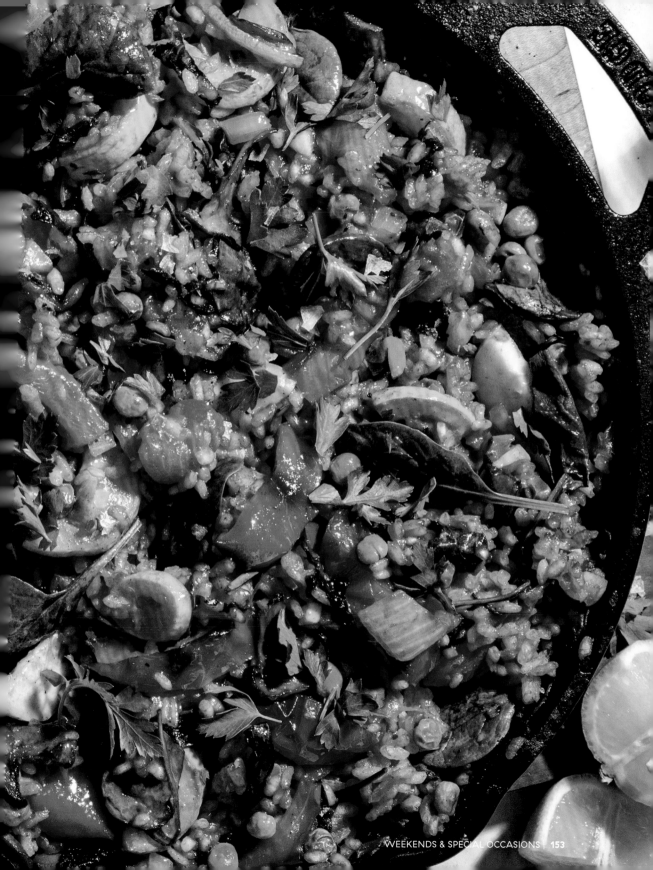

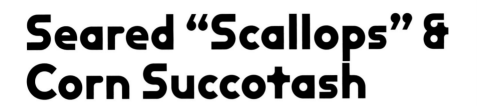

Seared "Scallops" & Corn Succotash

| 🍴 SERVES 4 | 🕐 TOTAL TIME: 50 MIN | |

In a dish that brings summer vibes to the table no matter the season, king trumpet mushrooms mirror the sweet, delicate flavor of sea scallops. Nestled into a colorful and crisp corn and snap pea succotash, this date-night-worthy dinner is sure to impress.

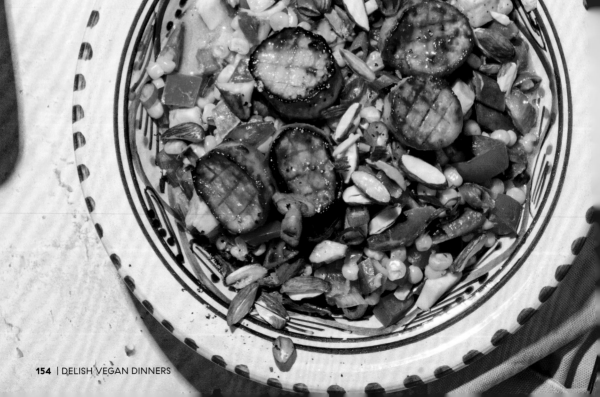

FOR THE "SCALLOPS"

2 tablespoons white miso

2 tablespoons mirin

2 tablespoons low-sodium soy
   sauce or tamari

6 large king trumpet mushrooms
   (1½ pounds), caps cut into small
   dice (1¼ cups), stems sliced
   crosswise into 1-inch-thick rounds

2 tablespoons canola oil

FOR THE SUCCOTASH

4 fresh ears of corn, shucked

1 tablespoon canola oil

1 tablespoon vegan butter

½ medium red onion, cut into
   small dice (1 cup)

1 medium red bell pepper,
   stemmed, seeded, and cut into
   small dice (1 cup)

3 cloves garlic, finely chopped

1 cup unsweetened almond milk

6 ounces snap peas, cut crosswise
   into thirds (1½ cups)

1 teaspoon toasted sesame oil

¼ teaspoon smoked paprika

Kosher salt

Freshly ground black pepper

2 green onions, chopped

½ cup thinly sliced almonds,
   toasted

1. Make "scallops": In a small bowl, whisk miso into mirin and soy sauce until smooth. Pour marinade into a shallow baking dish. Add mushroom stems to marinade, tossing to coat, then arrange stems with one cut side down. Marinate for at least 30 minutes and up to overnight in refrigerator, tossing scallops a few times.

2. Meanwhile, make corn succotash: Using a knife, remove kernels from corn (about 2½ cups kernels) and place in a bowl. Use back of knife to scrape any juice left on cob. Reserve juice separately from kernels; discard cobs.

3. For "scallops": Heat a large heavy-bottomed skillet over medium heat. Pour in oil and add "scallops" in a single layer, with one cut side down. Cook, turning once golden on first side, until both cut sides are golden, about 4 minutes. Remove to a plate.

4. Pour off any remaining oil in skillet and discard. Wipe skillet clean with paper towels.

5. For succotash: Return skillet to medium heat. Add canola oil and butter. When butter is melted, add onion and bell pepper. Cook, stirring occasionally, until starting to turn tender, about 2 minutes. Stir in chopped mushroom caps and garlic and cook, stirring occasionally, about 2 minutes more.

6. Add almond milk, corn kernels and reserved corn juice, snap peas, sesame oil, and paprika. Season with salt and pepper and stir to combine. Bring the mixture to a simmer.

7. Nestle scallops into corn mixture and cover skillet. Simmer for 5 minutes until scallops are tender throughout and corn and snap peas are crisp tender.

8. Spoon into bowls and top each bowl with green onions and almonds.

Eggplant "Steak" Frites with Chimichurri

 SERVES 4 **TOTAL TIME: 1 HR 40 MIN**

How do you successfully accomplish steak night without the beef? Sub in thick slices of creamy eggplant, then create a grilled mash-up of the classic French combo steak frites doused with an Argentine herb sauce, chimichurri.

FOR THE EGGPLANT "STEAKS"

1 large eggplant (about 1½ pounds), trimmed, cut lengthwise into ¼-inch slices

1½ teaspoons kosher salt

2 tablespoons extra-virgin olive oil

Freshly ground black pepper

FOR THE FRITES

4 medium russet potatoes, scrubbed and cut lengthwise into ½-inch wedges

1 teaspoon kosher salt

2 tablespoons extra-virgin olive oil

FOR THE CHIMICHURRI

1¼ cups packed fresh parsley leaves

3 tablespoons packed fresh oregano leaves

2 garlic cloves, chopped

⅓ cup extra-virgin olive oil

¼ cup red wine vinegar

½ teaspoon red pepper flakes

Kosher salt

1. Preheat grill or grill pan to medium-high. Generously season both sides of eggplant slices with salt. Arrange vertically in a colander set over a shallow bowl and let drain for 30 minutes. Rinse eggplant and pat dry. Brush both sides of eggplant with oil and season with salt and pepper.

2. Meanwhile, place potatoes in a large pot and add enough cold water to cover by 1 inch. Season the water with 1 teaspoon salt and place pot over high heat. Bring to a boil then reduce heat to medium and simmer until potatoes are just barely tender, about 5 minutes. Drain potatoes and transfer to a large bowl; pat dry. Toss with oil.

3. To make chimichurri, in a mini food processor, pulse parsley, oregano, and garlic until finely chopped. Transfer herb mixture into a small bowl and stir in olive oil, vinegar, red pepper flakes, and season with salt. Let sit so flavors can meld while cooking eggplant steaks and frites.

4. Grill eggplant and potatoes, turning halfway through, until eggplant is golden and tender inside, about 8 minutes, and potatoes are golden and crisp on outside and tender on inside, about 5 minutes. Remove each vegetable to a plate or tray as they are done. Season potatoes with salt as they come off grill.

5. Serve eggplant "steaks" with grilled frites and a generous dollop of chimichurri.

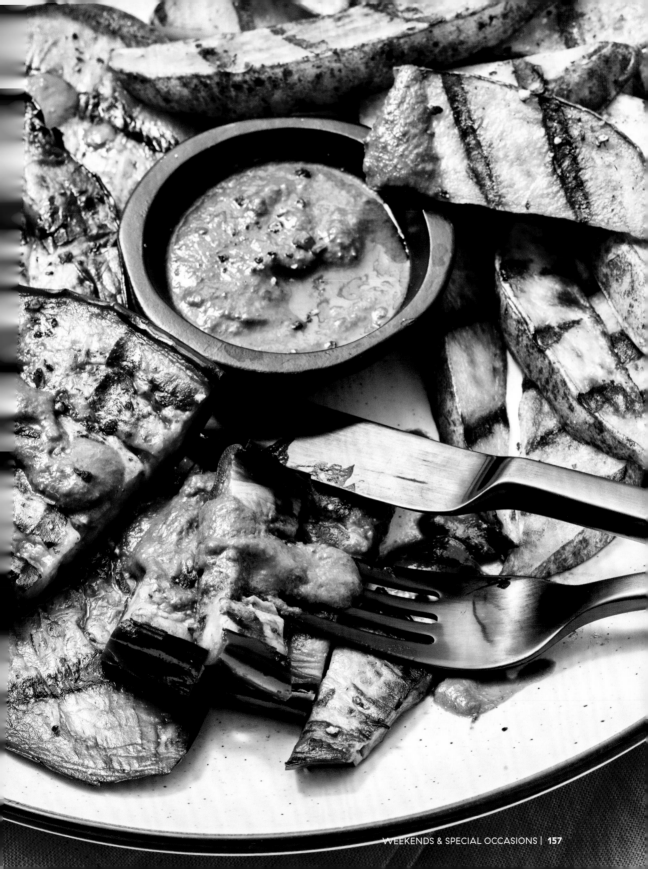

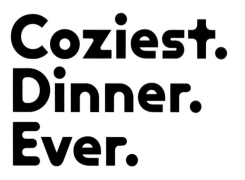

Coziest. Dinner. Ever.

There's no shortage of umami flavor in this **Mushroom Pot Pie**, thanks to a trifecta of funghi, both fresh and dry. A quick homemade veggie broth adds another layer of cozy flavor, and phyllo dough makes for a quick and shatteringly flaky crust.

TURN FOR THE RECIPE! →

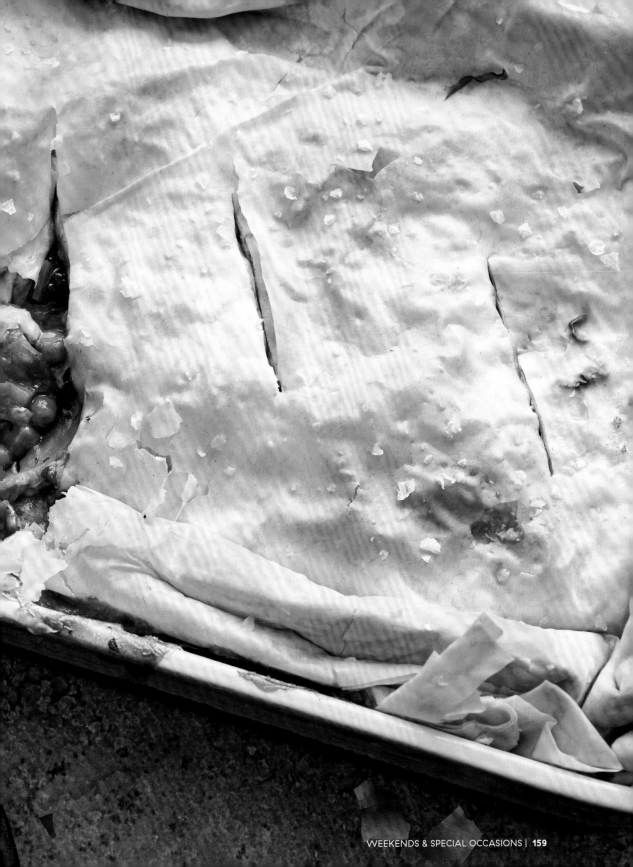

Mushroom Pot Pie

 SERVES 4–6　　　🕐 **TOTAL TIME: 2 HR 15 MIN**

1 medium yellow onion

2 medium carrots, peeled, divided

2 stalks celery, divided

3 garlic cloves, divided

3 sprigs thyme, divided

2 dried bay leaves

½ cup dried porcini mushrooms

Kosher salt

4 cups cold water

½ cup plus 2 tablespoons extra-virgin olive oil, divided, plus more if needed

8 ounces cremini mushrooms, quartered

Freshly ground black pepper

8 ounces shiitake mushrooms, sliced

2 teaspoons freshly chopped rosemary

2 teaspoons freshly chopped sage leaves

⅓ cup all-purpose flour

½ cup dry white wine

1 to 2 teaspoons low-sodium soy sauce

1½ cups fresh or frozen peas (if frozen, rinse and drain)

¼ cup freshly chopped parsley

8 (14x18-inch) sheets phyllo dough, defrosted if frozen

Flaky sea salt

1. Cut onion, 1 carrot, and 1 stalk of celery in half. Place one-half of each in a medium saucepan. Crush 1 clove garlic and add to pan along with 1 sprig of thyme, bay leaves, and porcini mushrooms. Season with salt, then cover with cold water. Bring mixture to a boil, then reduce heat to low simmer, and cover almost completely with a lid. Let simmer while you prep and cook pot pie filling.

2. Meanwhile, dice remaining onion, carrot, and celery. Peel and thinly slice remaining garlic cloves and pick leaves off remaining thyme sprigs, adding stems to broth pan and reserving leaves. Preheat oven to 400°F.

3. In a large skillet over medium-high heat, heat 1 tablespoon olive oil. Add cremini mushrooms, season with salt and pepper, and cook undisturbed for 4 minutes. Continue to cook, stirring occasionally, until mushrooms are slightly tender, 5 minutes. Transfer to a plate. Lower heat to medium, add another tablespoon olive oil, and repeat process with shiitake mushrooms. Transfer to same plate as creminis and wipe skillet clean.

4. Return skillet to medium heat, adding another tablespoon of oil. Add onions and carrots and season with salt and pepper. Cook, stirring occasionally, until onions are translucent and carrots are slightly tender, 4 to 5 minutes.

5. Add celery, sliced garlic, reserved thyme leaves, rosemary, and sage. Cook until garlic and herbs are fragrant, about 2 minutes, and season with salt and pepper. Turn off heat and remove skillet from burner.

6. Using tongs or a slotted spoon, remove and discard carrot, celery, onion, garlic clove, bay leaves, and thyme sprigs from broth. Strain broth into a large measuring cup, reserving porcini mushrooms. Transfer porcinis to cutting board and chop into small pieces. You should have around 3 cups of broth; if you have less than 3 cups, add cold water to stretch your broth to 3 cups.

7. Return skillet to medium heat, and when ingredients start to sizzle, add 2 more tablespoons olive oil and the flour. Cook, stirring constantly, until flour has darkened slightly in color and smells nutty, 2 to 3 minutes. (If your skillet is looking dry, add a splash of olive oil.)

8. Add white wine and half the prepared vegetable broth, stirring continuously to avoid lumps. Bring up to a simmer and cook until a thick gravy forms, about 3 minutes. Add remaining broth slowly, stirring continuously, until all is added and fully incorporated. Bring back to a boil and simmer until a velvety gravy forms, 8 to 12 minutes. To test gravy's thickness, stir it with a wooden spoon, then immediately trace a line on back of spoon with your finger, through gravy. If line fills in with liquid, gravy needs to simmer longer. If line remains visible, gravy is good to go!

9. Stir prepared cremini, shiitake, and porcini mushrooms into gravy. Taste for seasoning, then add soy sauce 1 teaspoon at a time, to taste. Remove from heat and stir in peas and parsley. Transfer mixture to a 9x13-inch baking dish.

10. Pour remaining 6 tablespoons olive oil into a small bowl. On a dry, clean surface, carefully unroll phyllo dough. Keep sheets covered with a kitchen towel while working with individual sheets. Place one sheet flat then use a pastry brush to coat entire sheet with a thin layer of olive oil. Place another sheet on top and repeat process.

11. When all 8 sheets are oiled and stacked, carefully transfer to baking dish. Any excess dough can be loosely folded around edges of pan. Sprinkle with flaky sea salt and use a sharp knife to cut 3 slits in crust.

12. Bake pot pie until phyllo is golden, 30 to 35 minutes. Let cool slightly before serving.

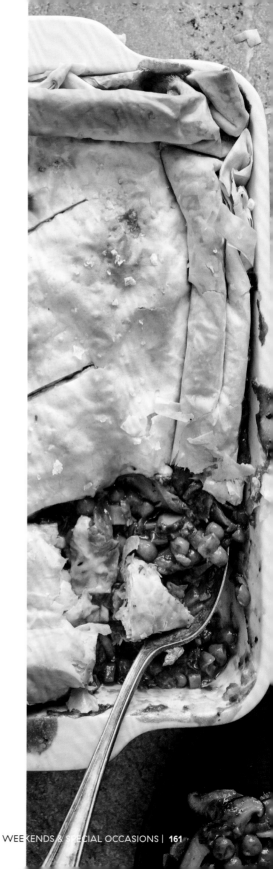

Spicy Fried "Chicken" Sandwich

 SERVES 4 | TOTAL TIME: 10 HR 30 MIN

We replicated fiery fried chicken with protein–packed tofu and added cornmeal to the batter for a bit of extra crunch.

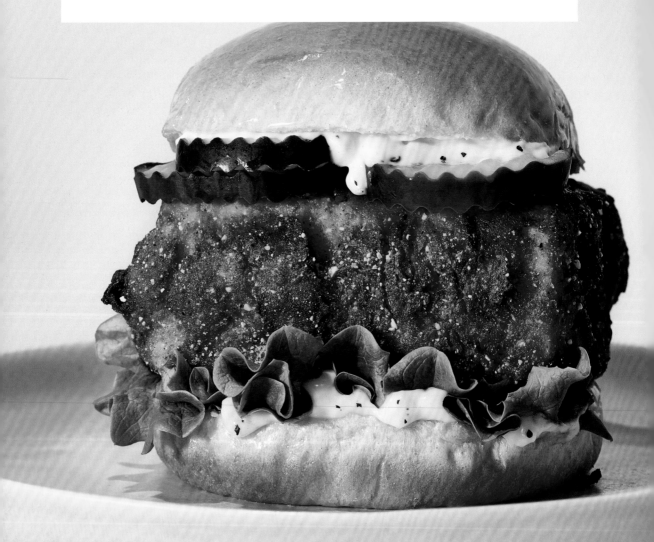

2 (14-ounce) blocks extra-firm
   tofu, excess liquid drained
¼ cup Dijon mustard
¼ cup brine from bread and butter
   pickles, plus pickle slices,
   for serving
¼ cup hot sauce, plus more
   for serving
2 tablespoons apple cider vinegar
1 cup all-purpose flour
½ cup finely ground cornmeal
1 tablespoon cornstarch
2 teaspoons chili powder
1½ teaspoons cayenne pepper
1 teaspoon onion powder
½ teaspoon baking powder
½ teaspoon garlic powder
½ kosher salt
Vegetable oil, for frying
4 fresh soft hamburger buns
4 leaves green leaf lettuce
Vegan mayonnaise

1. Arrange tofu in a single layer on a freezer-safe plate and cover with plastic wrap. Freeze solid, at least 5 hours and up to a month in advance.

2. Once frozen, let tofu defrost completely, 4 hours on counter or overnight in refrigerator. Drain excess water..

3. Arrange defrosted tofu in a single layer on a rimmed baking sheet lined with paper towels. Place a few more layers of paper towels and another rimmed baking sheet on top of tofu. Weight baking sheet with a few cookbooks. Let drain, changing paper towels when saturated with water, at least 1 hour or up to overnight in refrigerator.

4. When tofu is finished draining, make sandwich. In a shallow bowl, whisk together Dijon mustard, pickle brine, hot sauce, and vinegar. In another shallow bowl, whisk together flour, cornmeal, cornstarch, chili powder, cayenne pepper, onion powder, baking powder, garlic powder, and ½ teaspoon salt.

5. Cut each piece of tofu crosswise into 2 planks. Working with one piece at a time, coat tofu in dry mixture then dip in wet mixture. Return to dry mixture and repeat wet and dry one time.

6. Pour oil into a large cast-iron skillet until it comes ½ inch up side of skillet. Place over medium-high heat. When oil just starts to shimmer, reduce heat to medium and fry coated tofu in one batch, turning once, until golden on both sides, about 5 minutes per side. Transfer to a paper towel-lined plate to drain.

7. Spread garlic mayo on bottom of each bun. Top each with lettuce, a piece of fried tofu, and a small handful of pickles. Sandwich with top bun and serve.

PRO TIP!

If you're looking for texture similar to chicken, don't skip the freezing step. The texture of tofu transforms from firm and crumbly to chewy and meat-like.

Whole Roasted Cabbage

 SERVES 6   **TOTAL TIME: 1 HR 55 MIN**

Finally, a holiday centerpiece that *isn't* stressful to carve! This cabbage stunner is savory and smoky on the outside and juicy and sweet on the inside.

FOR THE CABBAGE

1 large head green cabbage
  (around 2 pounds)
3 tablespoons extra-virgin olive oil
1 tablespoon Dijon mustard
2 teaspoons maple syrup
1 teaspoon vegan Worcestershire
  sauce (optional)
½ teaspoon garlic powder
Kosher salt
Freshly ground black pepper
2 stalks celery, cut into quarters
2 medium carrots, peeled and cut
  into thirds
1 small yellow onion, quartered
1 tablespoon freshly chopped sage
1 tablespoon freshly chopped
  rosemary
1 tablespoon freshly chopped thyme
¾ cup low-sodium vegetable
  broth, divided
1 tablespoon freshly chopped
  parsley, for garnish

FOR THE GRAVY

¼ cup extra-virgin olive oil
½ onion, finely chopped
4 ounces cremini mushrooms,
  finely chopped
1 teaspoon freshly chopped sage
1 teaspoon freshly chopped
  rosemary
1 teaspoon freshly chopped thyme
Kosher salt
Freshly ground black pepper
3 tablespoons all-purpose flour
3 cups low-sodium vegetable
  broth

1. Preheat oven to 400°F. Cut stem off cabbage so it can sit flat.

2. Make sauce for cabbage: In a medium bowl, whisk together olive oil, mustard, maple syrup, Worcestershire sauce (if using), and garlic powder. Season with salt and pepper.

3. In a large bowl, combine celery, carrots, onion, oil, and chopped herbs. Season with salt and pepper and toss to coat.

4. Place vegetable mixture in a large, oven-safe skillet. Nestle cabbage in center, on top of vegetables, and brush all over with half of olive oil mixture. Pour ¼ cup broth into the bottom of skillet and cover cabbage with aluminum foil. Bake for 45 minutes.

5. When 45 minutes have passed, remove foil and brush with remaining olive oil mixture. Add remaining ½ cup broth and bake until cabbage is tender and slightly charred, 45 minutes more. (Pierce cabbage with a paring knife to check if it's ready.)

6. Meanwhile, make gravy: In a small saucepan over medium heat, heat oil. Add onion and cook, stirring until soft, 6 minutes. Stir in mushrooms and herbs and season with salt and pepper. Cook, stirring occasionally, until mushrooms are soft and golden, about 4 minutes. Stir in flour and cook 1 minute, then whisk in broth and bring mixture to a boil. Reduce heat to low and simmer until mixture has thickened to your desired consistency, 5 minutes. (Add more broth if desired.)

7. Slice cabbage into large wedges and serve with gravy. Garnish with parsley and serve hot.

Charred Lemon-Asparagus Risotto

 SERVES 4 | **TOTAL TIME: 50 MIN**

Take advantage of springtime's best produce with this surprisingly quick and simple risotto. The homemade Parm–esque topping is not to be missed.

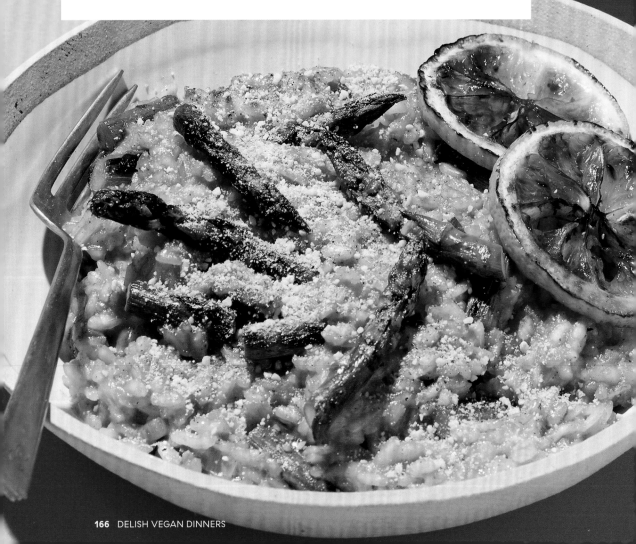

FOR THE RISOTTO

3 cups low-sodium vegetable broth

3 cups water

1 (1-pound) bunch asparagus, ends trimmed

1 lemon, thinly sliced into rounds, plus ¼ cup fresh lemon juice

½ large yellow onion, finely chopped

2 large shallots, finely chopped

3 tablespoons extra-virgin olive oil

1 teaspoon kosher salt, plus more for taste

3 cloves garlic, chopped

1½ cups arborio rice

2 tablespoons vegan butter

Freshly ground black pepper

FOR THE "PARMESAN" TOPPING

½ cup raw unsalted cashews

1 tablespoon nutritional yeast

¼ teaspoon garlic powder

¼ teaspoon onion powder

Kosher salt

1. Make risotto: In a medium pot, combine broth and water. Place over medium heat and bring to a low simmer. Reduce heat to low.

2. Meanwhile, heat a large straight-sided skillet over medium-high heat until very hot, about 2 minutes. Add half of asparagus in an even layer and cook, turning a few times, until crisp-tender and charred in places, about 4 minutes. Remove charred asparagus to a work surface and repeat with remaining asparagus.

3. Add lemon slices to skillet and cook, turning halfway through until lightly charred, about 2 minutes. Remove to work surface with asparagus.

4. Remove skillet from heat. Add onion and shallot and stir a few times. This mixture will char slightly almost immediately. Add oil and stir to coat.

5. Return skillet to medium heat. Season with a pinch of salt and cook, stirring occasionally, until onion mixture is softened, about 2 minutes. Add garlic and cook, stirring, until fragrant, about 2 minutes.

6. Stir rice into onion mixture and season with 1 teaspoon salt. Cook, stirring constantly, until rice is lightly toasted, about 2 minutes.

7. Pour lemon juice into rice mixture and bring to a boil. Cook, stirring constantly, until completely evaporated, about 1 minute.

8. Add a few ladles of warm broth mixture into skillet and cook, stirring until broth is absorbed. Continue to cook, adding a few ladles of broth as it is absorbed and stirring frequently, until rice is al dente, about 25 minutes.

9. Remove a few asparagus tips and set aside for garnish. Cut remaining asparagus into 1-inch pieces.

10. Make vegan Parmesan: In a food processor, pulse all ingredients with a pinch of salt until cashew is minced and everything is combined.

11. When rice is al dente, stir in butter, asparagus, and 1 tablespoon of vegan Parmesan until butter is melted and asparagus is warmed through. Season with salt and pepper. Garnish with remaining lemon slices and reserved asparagus. Sprinkle with more vegan Parmesan and serve warm.

Thank You

For Purchashing *Delish Vegan Dinners*

Visit our online store to find more great products from *Delish* and save **20% off your next purchase.**

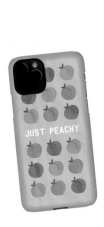
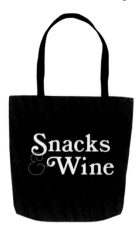
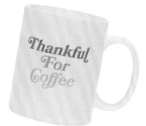

HEARST